HINDSIGHT:

What We Wish We Had Known At the Onset of Our Daughter's Sudden Descent into Anorexia

Lyn and Chris Ellis

DEDICATION

We dedicate this book to both our daughters:

Our older daughter, our hero, as she fights to recover the life
she so deserves and wants. Recovery from anorexia nervosa
is an epic battle. It requires dutiful vigilance
throughout the day, every day.
We love her more than all the stars in the night sky,
and are in constant awe of her will, her strength, her
self-determination, and focus;

and

Our younger daughter, for whom words cannot express our
bottomless love, gratitude, respect and admiration.
She went through every step of this with us and showed a
maturity, a steadfastness toward her older sister, and a depth of
caring well beyond her years.

ABOUT THE AUTHORS

Lyn and Chris Ellis are the parents of two young adult daughters struggling to make their way in a world where competition, and the pressure to perform and look perfect are amplified by social media. We have chosen to use pseudonyms and obscure certain details in order to protect the privacy for all concerned.

CONTENTS

ACKNOWLEDGMENTS

We cannot acknowledge everyone who helped us through our ED odyssey, but we wish to recognize those who provided crucial support, guidance and information at various points:

First and foremost, kudos to the Eating Disorder Resource Center of Silicon Valley (CA)—especially Janice Bremis, the EDRC's founder, whose vision and hard work created a bi-monthly parent support group that was enormously helpful in the early stages.

Evidence-based knowledge of eating disorder etiology – especially the understanding of genetic contributors and physiological factors – and effective treatment strategies – wouldn't be available if not for the enormous contributions by experts such as Dr. Walter Kaye, Dr. Daniel Le Grange, Dr. James Lock, and Dr. Janet Treasure, Dr. Kathleen Kara Fitzpatrick, and Dr. Pamela Carlton, among others. Though not our daughter's primary care providers, they took time from their harried schedules to selflessly respond to our desperate queries when we needed guidance, answers and reassurance. For this generosity to virtual strangers, we will forever be grateful.

We don't know where we'd be without the support and expertise of our dear (out-of-network) therapist, J. Cahill, who not only guided us toward being the best parents we could in the midst of our crisis, but who did so in spite of the many extra hours of paperwork and aggravation required of her in dealing with the insurance company, when agreeing to take us in as a "single case agreement."

Last, but by no means least, we deeply appreciate our "extended family" of friends and our siblings—whom we won't name so as to ensure everyone's privacy. We trust you know who you are! Your unwavering love, support and compassion sustained us as we struggled to find our way through the ED thicket. We would never have made it had we not been able to lean on you for so long, when we felt the weight of the world on our shoulders.

INTRODUCTION:
WHY WE DECIDED TO WRITE THIS BOOK

We love our two daughters more than life itself, and we would do anything in our power to protect them. If you are a parent looking at this book, you are—or suspect you may be—facing one of the most frightening and perplexing situations that can strike a family, just as we did at the end of 2009.

As soon as we knew what we were dealing with, we jumped into action. We spent every available moment mining for information on the Internet, contacting resources, calling university researchers, and reading books—many books (more than 50 in the first six months). These included clinical tomes describing the causes of *anorexia nervosa*, others presenting different treatment methodologies, some offering personal stories of being afflicted and in various stages of recovery, research abstracts—basically anything we could find. Sleep-deprived, but fiercely determined, we acquired knowledge and made connections—all of which seemed to take forever. Nothing happened fast enough to match the hurtling speed with which our daughter was falling down the rabbit hole.

Vital decisions had to be made along the way—about treatment teams and methods, what level of care was appropriate, whether our daughter should take a leave from school immediately or remain a student and address the problem simultaneously, whether professionals in her university town would be able to help, and so on. These decisions had to be made much sooner than we had the capacity to take in the necessary information—indeed, before we even knew enough to ask the questions that mattered.

Once we were beyond the critical stages of her disorder, we found ourselves wondering how things might have gone better for her had we known then what we know now. What agony could have been avoided or lessened? Which of the choices we made inadvertently prolonged the illness? What we know now is that the faster and more aggressively one attacks this illness the better the chances for full recovery. It's a race against time.

Could different choices, based on more comprehensive information, have decreased the opportunity for anorexia to carve habitual pathways in her brain? Put another way, did our decisions at various points—based on insufficient information and the urgency of the situation—allow the anorexia to take over in ways from which she may yet never fully recover? Is it our fault, to some extent, if she is unable to permanently beat this thing, simply because we didn't know enough, in spite of our best efforts and intentions?

In hindsight, we feel that most of the professionals who treated our daughter during her critical phase were not aggressive enough, in spite of our constantly imploring them to do more, faster. Most seemed annoyed with our involvement, regarding it as an intrusion into their professional territory; some assumed that our intensity after she got sick was how we must have been as parents prior to her illness, thereby extrapolating that her developing this illness was a rebellion against our control. Nothing could be further from the truth.

But how could we prove that to people who didn't know us prior to this crisis? They are the "experts" after all, so no matter how much we cited recent research (which some of them weren't even familiar with!) that suggest refeeding must take place over a long enough period before someone struggling with anorexia can grasp and incorporate psychotherapeutic insights, and no matter how many times we argued that *we* are the "experts" on our daughter, in their minds we were just crazed parents who lacked the academic standing to justify our expressing ideas and asking questions along the way.

Our frustration with them and the roadblocks we encountered, and their displeasure with us and our involvement, prompted them to perform what is known as a "parentectomy"— in which they colluded with our daughter's illness to exclude us from providing or receiving information about her health or care. When we called them on it, they said this was essential for her recovery, but we felt they were caving in to her illness. She was extremely angry with us for "interfering" with her "right" to manage (or mismanage, from our perspective) her health, and they used her anger as evidence that we were interfering with her process of individuating and growing up.

We had no power to fight their decision to exclude us, thanks to HIPAA privacy laws. Within months of our being cut out of the picture—in spite of our many (futile) attempts to get information from the treatment team, and in spite of them promising they wouldn't let her fall through the cracks—our daughter's weight plummeted, her depression, anxiety and compulsive behavior around food skyrocketed, her behavior around us and around food became increasingly irrational and possibly psychotic—all as a result of her ongoing semi-starvation. She ended up having to return to residential treatment for a second time. Given her heart rate and other physical measures, it may have been just in the nick of time. We were furious that the teams let her get so ill before recommending a higher level of care.

Had we known more about the various modes of treatment, had we understood that "professionals" don't necessarily incorporate research findings into their treatment protocols, and had we understood the nature of loopholes in this illness, we would never have put our daughter's life in their hands. We would have known the importance of interviewing these providers and dismissing them in search of others who understand the need to tie up loopholes (not create them), and who would align with parents against the illness, not collude with the illness against the parents. Treatment professionals will often mistake the anger a child displays toward parents in the acute stages of the illness as a normal part of adolescent development, seeing it as a healthy expression of independence, when it is actually the illness *fiercely trying to maintain its hold on the child.* Given that eating disorders develop most often during adolescence, one can understand mistaking the source of the anger.

Had we also understood that the older books describing eating disorders were written prior to advances in the study of genetics and the development of technologies to see inside the brain, and prior to recent research on effective treatment methods, we would have known that many of the theories used to explain the causes and treatment of anorexia were based on outmoded or untested hypotheses. The researchers and practitioners who stay current on scientific research now agree that eating disorders, including anorexia nervosa, are **bio-psycho-social** illnesses. Because we didn't know better at the outset, we relied on treatment providers who viewed the illness as an emotionally-based disorder. Effective treatment means incorporating *evidence-based* research results. This requires many treatment professionals to change their operating paradigms, especially those who developed their beliefs and practices in the era when scientific research data was not available.

If we'd had accurate information up front, how much agony could our daughter have been spared? How much better would her chances be now for full recovery? We will never know for sure, because life doesn't give the opportunity to replay actual scenarios with the benefit of hindsight, but what we do know is that more knowledge might have allowed us to avoid many pitfalls. We sincerely hope the information and resources presented in this book will help guide you on the rock-strewn path of this insidious disorder. Becoming knowledgeable will help reduce your distress and decrease your child's pain, and maybe even save her life.

PART ONE: WHAT IS IT?, WHAT CAUSES IT?, AND WHAT ARE THE ESTABLISHED LEVELS OF CARE?

CHAPTER ONE: A BOLT OF LIGHTNING STRIKES AND SHE SPLITS INTO TWO

Anorexia struck our family like a bolt of lightning. Our daughter's descent down the rabbit hole was sudden and horrific. We didn't see it coming; How could we? Why *would* we?

We'd always been a close family, our two daughters always our first priority. We chose to have Lyn be a stay-at-home mom, to provide the anchor we feel children need, to have a more relaxed environment in which to raise a family, and to have more time together to allow for the development of relationships. We made every attempt to encourage the kids to develop their own interests, separate from ours, so they could feel individually accomplished, and not competitive with us in any way. As they grew, we allowed them many freedoms and responsibilities other parents we knew were not allowing, in the belief that it would help them strengthen their wings before launching from the nest.

When our older daughter went off to college, we reigned in our natural inclination to initiate communication with her too often, so as to give her the chance to determine when she wanted to talk with us. We didn't want to hover. We were thrilled when she called or wanted to Skype with us; when we did speak, nothing in those conversations suggested she wasn't thriving. We didn't notice any storm clouds on the horizon.

To this day, we don't know when or how her descent began, precisely, and we can only guess as to the environmental factors that may have contributed. Had her eating disorder started during that first fall when she went away? Had the physiological consequences of malnutrition already begun to take effect when she came home over Christmas break, even though we couldn't see any difference on the outside and we didn't discern any behavioral clues right away? Or did it begin only in the two weeks prior to the outbreak, when we witnessed behavior resembling burnout and mild depression—at which time we had no way of knowing she hadn't been eating? Was the onset that sudden?

She returned home during Christmas vacation from a very busy first quarter of college, worn out but seemingly happy. Concerned that for several weeks she'd been experiencing what felt like hot flashes, we arranged an appointment with her doctor for the day she came home. Her physician found nothing amiss. (She hadn't lost any weight at that point.) The doctor didn't know what to make of the hot flashes, as there was no indication by other measure that anything was wrong. We all shrugged it off, attributing it to stress.

She had come home early on December 12th, stumbling off the Greyhound, groggy from the all-night bus ride. Mom knew just the kind of comfort food that would lull her back into a well-earned and well-deserved morning nap: my nutrition-laden version of miso soup, stocked with wakame, veggies, potatoes and an egg. This had been a favorite of hers for years, and she knew she'd have been yearning for home-cooked food after enduring cafeteria food the past several months. She dug in, happily.

The next two weeks, nothing seemed hugely out of the ordinary, at least with regard to food. We both worked during the day, and she was sleeping a lot, which wasn't unreasonable given that she'd burned herself out by the demands of that first academic quarter; she succumbed to the sublime pleasure of sleeping at home, in her own bed. We didn't eat breakfast together those first two weeks, due to our differing schedules, but we managed several family dinners. All seemed relatively normal.

The second week she was home, a pall crept over our home: Even after plenty of rest, our daughter lacked her normal, pre-holiday cheer; she did not display her usual get-up-and-go energy that we knew so well from the past: She'd always been the one to instigate ritual holiday shopping for the family, but now her joie-de-vivre was muted. She became increasingly reclusive over the next few weeks, staying in bed and watching TV reruns or movies on her computer, unresponsive to offers to get up and out of the house. We glanced at each other, shrugged helplessly, and when we had a few moments to confer privately, we concluded she was probably just burned out—plus we knew she was feeling disconnected from her boyfriend and the few high school friends who were in town but not in touch. Her friendships had always been important, yet so complicated. Those complications tainted her high school years, particularly her senior year. Now, old friends weren't calling much; it didn't appear she was reaching out to them, either.

We avoided asking her directly what was going on, as we'd been singed by her fiery retorts far too often before. We knew that asking too much or too frequently was something she experienced as an intrusion into her closely guarded private life. Though it was not the way either of us were, or how we wanted our relationship with her to be, we had long ago learned she was different from us; we reasoned that good parenting required honoring who she was.

During the week leading up to Christmas, then, we had no idea anything was amiss. Normal moodiness, burnout from studying, the usual frustrations with friends: we tried to put the best spin on her behavior and demeanor that we could. Fast forward to Christmas Eve, when life with our daughter abruptly spun wildly out of control. Like on a Joy Wheel at the amusement park, accelerating at a dizzying speed, we were losing our grip—only there was no padding to cushion our fall, just a bottomless chasm that we were being flung into, with nothing to grab hold of.

Christmas Eve dinner in our home has always been untraditional, but also something special to us: a hearty soup of vegetable, bean and pasta, topped with cheesy bread in the style of French onion soup. An easy, simple, healthy, warm, homemade, comfort-inducing, one-course dinner. But this year, I (Lyn) instinctively knew (without knowing *why*) not to put the bread on the soup, instead placing it separately on a plate so that each person could choose to add it or not. Our daughter took no cheesy bread; this was unusual, but we sloughed it off—assuming perhaps she wanted to keep fit as she had recently earned a spot on the university's club volleyball team. We even recall her saying, at one point, that she wanted to lose a little weight so that she could jump higher (which didn't seem unreasonable at the time, although in retrospect we recall wondering why jumping would seem so critical to a volleyball *setter*).

Washing the dishes later, I noticed that when she cleared her place at the table, instead of putting her bowl in the sink, she left it rather conspicuously on the counter where one couldn't help noticing it. At the time, I was mildly annoyed at the lack of follow through, wishing we had been better about getting the girls to wash their own dishes over the years. But, as things unfolded, it later struck us as somehow deliberate—some part of her *wanted us to notice* that she hadn't eaten the noodles, not a single one as far as we could tell. Abstaining from cheesy toast was one thing, but this is a kid who had LOVED noodles all her life—whose first word for food, in fact, was "noo-noos."

We didn't comment at the time, but in hindsight that has come to seem a pivotal moment—signaling a turning point in her relationship with food, and in our relationship with her. And it became clear, as events unfolded over the next two days or so, that it must have been her way, even if on a subconscious level, of trying to communicate that she was losing control—or rather, in the anorexic's twisted logic, desperately trying to regain the control she felt she had lost along the way. Was this a cry for help? A defiant slap in our faces? Not that she would characterize it that way, but a mom *knows* what a mom knows. Call it intuition. Call it knowledge gained from the accumulation of all those years together. But I *knew* something was terribly wrong.

The following morning—Christmas Day—the mood in the house was distressingly unfestive. We had become hostage to some uninvited, unseen

8

visitor; an intruder had invaded our sanctuary. Christmas morning in our home normally involved the kids getting up early and eagerly, happily joining me in the kitchen to cook something special and fun. An air of excitement and anticipation had always filled the house along with the aroma of pumpkin bread and mulled cider. But not this year; the train had come off the tracks. Our daughters did *not* appear on the landing in their p.j.s to gaze down on the tree and the mound of presents; in fact they did not join us until nearly 1:30 that afternoon, and only then after we'd called them downstairs. Bizarre— and worrisome, to say the least.

Alone in the kitchen, I made pumpkin spice pancakes, sausage and fruit for a late brunch—pretty limited fare as holiday meals go, and she remembers thinking there was no point in putting butter or syrup on the table—certainly not if our daughter had disdained pasta, cheese and bread the night before. When the girls finally responded to our calls to come downstairs, the older one sat at the table with furrowed brow, disengaged from the family, seemingly retreated to some dark place inside. In a sullen trance, she picked her way through a few small pancakes, and nothing more. We had no idea of the fierce, internal battle consuming her.

Details of gift giving that Christmas are lost to memory, but we distinctly recall the absence of any special holiday feeling, any sense of joy and togetherness in the occasion. Our time together didn't last long; as soon as we finished opening presents, she burst from the room, announcing that she couldn't believe what a pig she had been for eating so many pancakes. Dumbstruck, we cast worried glances at one other, and we had no idea what to do.

She stayed in her room the rest of the day, and tensions increased. She made only one appearance in the evening, when she left to meet her boyfriend for coffee. We sat stunned and saddened by the weird, disturbing scenario unfolding in front of us.

The next day, she again slept until 1:30, which worried us greatly because we now knew she hadn't eaten anything in 24 hours, not since the pancakes from the day before. Lunch on this day was homemade hummus and carrots — always a favorite in the past—and once it became clear she wasn't joining us at the table, we asked her sister to take some up to her so she would have *something* while she lay in bed. Not that we wanted her to stay isolated like that, but we figured at least this way she could receive a modicum of nutrition while she wrestled with whatever demon had taken hold of her.

The offer of hummus triggered a Vesuvius-like explosion that destroyed what fragile peace remained in our home. She came barreling out of her room, tray in hand, yelling—as if possessed and strangling on her own words, in a voice we barely recognized: "Why are you doing this to me? Why are you trying to make me eat? Why are you CONTROLLING me? I am not hungry. I don't want to eat." The force of her vitriol pinned us to the wall, rendering us speechless. The dragon withdrew to its room, and when we peeled ourselves off the wall, we staggered around like zombies scorched by a fireball.

Somehow, we had to pull ourselves together, try to make sense of what was happening. A close friend from abroad was coming to dinner the following evening, so a batch of prep work needed to be performed in the kitchen. We had planned a nice American meal for our guest: steak (a rare treat in our house) with Roquefort sauce; broiled garlic potatoes, caramelized onions, mushrooms in a wine glaze. Still stunned and growing increasingly frightened by (among other things) our daughter not having eaten a single morsel in well over 24 hours, we focused on preparing for our visitor. Never far from our minds was the thought that she's got to eat *something*, but what, and how? Clearly, she didn't want anything from me; she thought I was trying to control her! But whatever was making her so crazed, it couldn't be as strong as her lifelong love of udon soup . . . could it? Knowing she'd be less likely to accept it if openly offered, we slipped in and placed it on the desk in her room when she went to take shower. Several hours later, we found the tray on the bathroom counter. Not a word had been exchanged about it or anything else, for that matter. The broth, with no calories, had been consumed but not a single noodle, vegetable or bean. Our anxiety by then was spiraling to a fever pitch.

Dinnertime came and she abruptly emerged from her room frantic, saying she had unbearable cabin fever, and practically begged me to drive downtown with her. Though whipped from the emotional upheaval, combined with the hours prepping the following night's dinner, this was clearly a time of need, and she wanted my company. Out we went.

Our daughter has always been a critical driver, vocal about every mistake other drivers make. But on this occasion the expression of her anger was so intense that she seemed possessed. I placed my hand on her arm, and took a chance to express my deep concern: "Honey, what's going on? You seem so depressed…. So angry." Jerking away her arm, she burst into tears and blurted out, "Can't you tell? I have no friends. I hate this town." I said we'd noticed she hadn't been calling her friends, but that we felt something bigger was going on: I said we feared she was depressed and that maybe, perhaps, she was anorexic, given how little she'd eaten the past couple of days. She acknowledged being depressed (a huge admission for her), but the mention of anorexia completely unraveled her.

How could we have known that was NOT the thing to say to someone under the sway of anorexia? We didn't even know what anorexia was, after all, other than an extreme quest for thinness—a diet taken too far, perhaps. We had not yet learned that anorexia is a *psychiatric illness*, with severe physical consequences, and that it has the highest mortality rate of any mental disorder. We had no clue about its egosyntonic nature, in which the sufferer's identity is deeply entwined in the beliefs that underscore it and the behaviors that manifest it—in short, to people victimized by anorexia, the notion of letting go of it is akin to losing their entire sense of self? Who knew that there is an illness in which the sufferer finds such comfort in it that they protect it with whatever means they can create? Particularly in the acute stages of anorexia, sufferers hold on tenaciously to the disorder, defying logic and common sense (to say nothing of the entreaties of friends and family trying to keep them from self-destructing).

My expression of concern that our daughter might be anorexic caused her to flip out, screaming that she didn't invite company for the drive to town so they could argue; she started to turn the car around, intent on taking me home so she could go shopping on her own. I begged her not to; she went along but didn't say another word the rest of the time they were out. I couldn't cajole her into engaging at all. It was horrible. Our daughter later persisted in characterizing that expression of concern as "a fight."

When they got home, it was well past dinnertime, and I implored Chris to go upstairs and persuade her to eat something, since she'd made it clear she wouldn't accept a thing from me. Chris was more passive than me in most situations, usually taking time to ponder situations before acting, and this was no exception. I made it clear there wasn't time for contemplation; the urgency in my voice unnerved him. He realized he had to get involved, *now*.

Some time passed, and I was relieved when Chris reported that she had agreed to have some soup if it was brought up to her. Phew, we thought. Maybe this had been just some weirdness that would blow over. I put together a tray of soup, a small bowl of popcorn with hot sauce (which is how she'd told us she and her college roommate liked it), and a cup of tea. Encouraged by this turn of events, I entered her room, tray in hand, and when I put the tray down, she again yelled that she was NOT going to eat. Shocked and confused, I told her what Dad had said she'd said, and she retorted—again in that derisive, dismissive voice: "I only *said* that to get him to go away." She didn't eat any of it.

Desperate and panicky, I went into high gear, spending much of that night searching the Internet. *Was* she anorexic? What *is* anorexia? Had she gone mad? Were we witnessing a mental breakdown, a psychotic episode? If it was anorexia, what had caused it? What behaviors are associated with it? Where could we go to get help? What kind of help was available (on a holiday weekend, no less!)? What were we supposed to do, especially with her expected return to college (300 miles away) in less than a week?

Everything I read that night about typical anorexia behaviors coincided perfectly (and frighteningly) with everything we'd been experiencing. Even more unnerving, perhaps, was what we read about personality traits and cognitive styles common to anorexics. Common personality traits include a tendency toward perfectionism, obsessiveness, and anxiety, being risk averse and introverted. Cognitively, those who become anorexic are typically very intelligent, quick to judge, exhibit rigid "black and white" thinking, have a difficulty in set shifting (the ability to change cognitive strategies as needed), and have a tendency to catastrophize even common events, among other things. What unnerved us is that the description applied 100% to our daughter!

How could the writers be describing our daughter so accurately? Why had we never heard that these characteristics are the ingredients that comprise a virtual recipe for the development of anorexia? Yes, our daughter had always been intense, moody, risk averse, introverted—all of it. Yes, she pushed herself to the max in everything she did, becoming increasingly perfectionistic and obsessive, especially during her last year of high school when trying to complete those damn college-application essays. How many times did we tell her they were "good enough," that it didn't need another edit at 2 a.m., that what she really needed was a good night's sleep? When exactly did she start bemoaning her 4.4 grade-point-average compared to her classmates' 4.8 GPA's? Our stomachs were knotted and churning, sick at the realization of what we were now dealing with.

Early the next morning before anyone was up, I texted our daughter's boyfriend—a first-time-ever intrusion into her private relationship, done so only out of desperation. She told him she needed to speak with him urgently, but privately. We needed information, and we needed it now. She asked him: Did our daughter seem different lately? How was she around food and mealtimes? He said she was acting weird, aloof, moody. He was frustrated that they were no longer able to go to their favorite haunts to eat. She was always telling him she'd just eaten with us and wasn't hungry. (She'd been telling us the same thing, we knew—that she wasn't hungry because she'd just gone out to eat with him.) This is classic anorexic lying, as we later learned. He went on to say she'd become emotionally distant. They were having no fun.

He mentioned plans to take her to lunch that day, and they actually went out for Vietnamese noodle soup. I pretended not to notice when she returned with a take-out container of leftovers. As soon as she left the room, I opened the container and saw that it was full . . . of noodles, her longtime favorite fare.

When she returned from a trip to the mall after that measly lunch, we sat down to the steak dinner for our out-of-town guest and several friends. I started serving everyone, as was customary especially with guests, and when it came to our daughter's plate, she gestured for me not to put too much on. So I dished up about a quarter of everyone else's serving, even the onions and mushrooms, which were among her favorites. Little did we know that would be the last meal any of us would serve her for a very long time.

After dinner, she went immediately to the bathroom. I knew enough by then to be concerned that our daughter was planning to purge what she had just eaten; she was in the guest bathroom an unusually long time, and finally I excused myself from the table and quietly approached the bathroom door. I couldn't hear anything unusual, but knocked on the door, mocking surprise to learn the bathroom was occupied. The not-so-subtle intent was to let her know we were on to her. She said she was washing her face— which I knew wasn't the case, as our daughter had never before used that bathroom (which she hated) for her face-washing ritual. She only washed her face upstairs where all her supplies are, before she turns in for the night. This was a pathetic attempt to cover up something. And yet we'd never known her to lie before. Pretending not to be in distress, I returned to the table to try to socialize with our guests. When she returned a bit later, our daughter wrapped herself in a blanket and avoided eye contact with everyone. Some dark force had taken over her soul.

My friend and I had made plans months prior to go to a nearby resort town for a couple of nights —a Christmas treat. Naturally, I was in a quandary about what to do. Feeling there was little to be accomplished by staying home while our daughter's hostility was directed principally at her, knowing that we wouldn't be able to get through to professionals to get advice (thanks to the holidays), and not wanting to disappoint the friend by bailing out on their plan, I decided to go. Two days away would afford an opportunity to think things over, to figure out a strategy to deal with this, and might ease the tension for our daughter. I implored our other daughter to keep a surreptitious eye on her sister's food behavior, so we could get a sense of what transpired while I was gone. (It turned out she ate only one meal each day, and nothing with significant caloric content. This marked our unofficial confirmation of the anorexia diagnosis.)

When it was time to return, I called saying I'd say be home in two hours. We were greeted at the door by the aroma of freshly baked chocolate cake; feigning an air of normalcy, our daughter said she had made it for us. She immediately asked me to make the frosting. I wasn't much in the mood, being tired from the trip and still needing to entertain her friend, but I gave in to her pleas, only later realizing that it was her way of keeping me in the kitchen so I would witness her eating, as if to say, "See, Mom, all is normal." While I made frosting, our daughter took out some leftover salad and ate it along with a bite of a Hershey bar. But then she headed straight for the bathroom again, and was there for longer than normal, and I of course suspected purging. When she came out, she wouldn't touch the cake she'd just made. (I had recently read about how not eating what one has cooked for others is typical anorectic behavior. Seeing this only served to deepen our conviction about what we were dealing with.)

Worse yet, a short time later I opened one of the normally well-organized kitchen cabinets to find plates and bowls strewn about in the most helter-skelter fashion. I knew instinctively who had done this, and immediately got the underlying message: NOTICE me, HELP me, *DO SOMETHING*. Our daughter seemed to be losing her grip. The disheveled cabinet seemed a physical representation, a metaphor, for what was going on in her head. It also occurred to me that this could be our daughter's subconscious way to pick a fight. I could easily envision what would transpire if I reacted to the mess in the cabinet: it would validate her conviction that I was a "controlling bitch," etc. Case closed. I avoided the confrontation, and was heart-broken.

We didn't see our daughter at all the next day. She was asleep when I left the house, and she was at her boyfriend's house by the time I returned. Assuming she was going to be out with him that evening, and with Chris and our other daughter at different holiday gatherings, I decided to go to a movie with her aunt who lives nearby. I called our daughter to check in, finding out that she would be home by 6:00 p.m. and was quite surprised when she said *she didn't want to be alone that evening* (something she rarely expressed). So I happily shifted plans, asking her if she'd like to come along for the movie. She said yes, but only tentatively, as clearly something else was going on because she adamantly—vehemently, even—opposed seeing any film that was suggested, even the movies I was sure would appeal to her. When they couldn't agree on a movie, I suggested she rent a DVD that she liked and they could all watch it together at home. Again, she reluctantly agreed to this but it became clear she had little interest or enthusiasm for the idea. When she got to Blockbuster, she called in the midst of a major tizzy, upset that she had forgotten her money. When she got home, frazzled and without any movie, she said she couldn't stand the idea of watching anything, after all.

Confrontation: Right or wrong?

With the mood that evening having deteriorated precipitously, I knew we'd have to say something soon. But we also anticipated that it would be a battle of her perception against ours (a not uncommon pattern, especially between her and me even in the best of times). Knowing she would hate an intervention, it nevertheless seemed the most effective way of tackling this situation, given how little time we had left before vacation ended and she was back at school. We just didn't have time to get sidetracked with detours and deflected argumentation, such as endless arguments over perceptions. So, while she was at the video store, I called the boyfriend to ask if he'd be okay if I brought up his concerns. I also asked her aunt to stay and be part of the confrontation. We hoped their participation would reinforce our perceptions. *We all saw what was happening*; how could she dispute it?

When she returned from the video store, agitated and with no video, we sat her down and came right out with it: "We are desperately concerned about the depression we are witnessing, and your anger, and all of us—Dad, your sister, your aunt, and your boyfriend—everyone you've interacted with this vacation is deeply concerned that you have become anorexic." She immediately receded as if into a dark cave, began furiously texting on her cell phone, and bolted from the room and the house; she drove off with the car and was gone the rest of the evening. We sat, stunned and bewildered, like the survivors of a tornado that just blasted through our small town. Nothing like this had ever happened before in our family. She had been a sometimes testy teenager, but had never bolted from a scene (she was far more likely to fight through an argument to the bitter end!), and she had never taken the car without asking, nor had she ever left without telling us when she'd be home.

Frantic, I enlisted Chris's help the moment he got home from work: Find her, talk to her, cajole her into coming home. He did locate her, and she told him she'd return only if he could get me to promise not to talk about it; he agreed to that on my behalf—anything to get her back in the house. She proceeded to try to convince him that she didn't have a problem and told him she'd prove it by showing how normal she could be around food for her remaining days at home.

I was outraged that Chris would take her at her word, for believing things might be okay, after all we'd been experiencing. Couldn't he see that anyone—even an anorexic—could do *anything* to prove a point if only for a few days?

As it turned out, though, she couldn't do even that much. Her best effort to show us she was okay was to consume a fraction of what a static body needs to maintain equilibrium. It was doubly frightening that she thought such minimal intake would somehow convince us. Was she in the midst of a psychotic episode? Was she delusional? Trying to effect normalcy, her behavior became more bizarre, her actions even more erratic.

Virtually overnight, we were not allowed to offer her anything—not even a cup of her favorite hot tea, a ritual in our home for years. Mistakenly thinking that surely she might accept something with zero calories, I brought her a cup of tea. Her reaction was instantaneous and vicious, announcing loudly with astonishing candor: "I'm not going to drink it *because it came from YOU*!" I tried responding with simple logic and compassion that it contained no calories, and that her body needed at least minimal hydration. She defiantly held her ground.

I left the room, again stunned and bewildered. A half hour later, she stormed into our room, slammed the empty cup on my desk, and said, "There, I drank it!" Was she angrily conceding that we had won this skirmish? Was she mad at herself for being too weak to have refused it? We were more befuddled and terrified than ever.

That was between Christmas and New Year's in 2009. I was on the Internet for several days, at all hours, sending emails, making phone calls, trying to connect with someone—anyone—who might be able to provide professional insight or answers to our many questions. She couldn't even get a live voice on the other end of the phone: Everyone was on vacation! And we were scheduled to drive her back to school at the end of the New Year's weekend in just a few days, to start her next quarter's classes that Monday.

First, however, we had to figure out whether we could allow her to return to school under these circumstances. She was adamant about going back. We hadn't yet come to understand that this was her ED (eating disorder) "voice" speaking through her, demanding privacy and autonomy; obviously, if she could get away from us, she could continue listening to and obeying that voice, which was dragging her down into the depths of what we now understand is among the most insidious disorders known in the science of mental health.

Without professional input, we struggled mightily with the decision about school. Keeping her at home was a risky option: We didn't know where or to whom we were supposed to send her for help, how much time it would take each day or each week, or how we would contain this human tornado when she'd made it clear she could not abide being in our town where she had no social life and felt controlled and blackmailed by our overriding her decisions. What if her depression or anger toward us got worse, and made it impossible for her to focus on getting help? What if she became suicidal? She had much to live for and motivate her at school: her studies, new friendships, the upcoming volleyball season, and more. What if those were the things that could help elevate her out of her depression, and eventually *get her to eat*? If we were, indeed, part of the problem (as the first therapist we encountered by phone suggested unsubtly and without irony), maybe it would be best if our daughter *were* back at school, and out from under us.

I continued calling clinics and providers (both local and in her college town) who listed themselves as ED specialists. She left voicemails at the university's Student Health Services, asking what services they offered and what sort of outreach they would perform when informed a student is in trouble or suffering in some way but not willing to seek help because she's in denial. I found a list of therapists in that school town, and left messages on all their answering machines. Meantime, a friend called his brother who is a well-known psychiatrist, who was gracious enough to get off the ski slope where he was vacationing and phone us back to help us problem solve. As grateful as we were for his input, that conversation proved inconclusive since he was not a specialist in ED, nor was he familiar with experts in the field. We remained at a loss about what to do, and time was ticking.

18

We finally heard from just one therapist that holiday weekend, located in the college town, who said she would be willing to meet with us on Monday, if we decided to deliver our daughter to school. That was our first, faint ray of hope, but it was enough to hint that we might yet save our daughter even as we allowed her, against our better judgment, to return to school.

Our daughter was predictably repulsed and derisive when we presented to her what we regarded as our most reasonable, compromise offer. First, we pointed out that the safest thing for her was to stay home and figure out how to get help she needed once the professionals had returned from the holiday break.

Second, we knew how much school meant to her and we wanted to *honor her need for autonomy*, so we would (reluctantly) allow her to return for winter quarter. However, her return was conditional on entering and committing to stay in treatment, even if it meant reducing her course load and other commitments at school. As part of this deal, I would accompany her back to school and help get her team of treatment professionals set up (it was clear she wouldn't, or couldn't, do this herself, in the state she was in). It was also made clear that I wouldn't leave unless and until she felt comfortable that we had established a reliable safety net.

She exploded in outrage. She shouted that she wouldn't drive back down with me (even though less than a week prior—before all this started—she had sweetly asked me to drive her back because she hated the all-day train ride). We felt we were bending over backwards by agreeing to let her go back; her interpretation was that she was being given an ultimatum—she audaciously claimed that we were *blackmailing* her by threatening to withhold college funding if she didn't go along. She was flummoxed that we were willing to stare down the ED devil from whose lair she now glared at us. At this point she hadn't admitted to us (much less to herself) that she even had a problem. (The inability to detect or feel that there is a problem is a symptom of the illness, actually, and we describe this in detail a little further on.). At any rate, since she felt she was fine, she did not accept or appreciate our right to fight for her life. From her perspective (warped as a result of the semi-starvation), we were interfering with her right to self-determination.

As we write this, it has been approximately two years since this monster invaded our home. We've gone through hell and back, and while our daughter is clearly on a path of recovery, we don't know how soon she'll "arrive" or where this will all lead. We know that recovery is neither a straight trajectory nor a sure thing. No matter how well she is doing, in the back of our minds is the keen awareness that the "cure" for this malady could yet take us down a long, torturously winding, and expensive road.

Everything we've read confirms that the chances for recovery from ED increase dramatically the sooner those afflicted receive aggressive treatment. Did we intervene quickly enough? Were the treatments she received effective enough? Did the choices we made along the way (and were sometimes forced to make by timing, or limited knowledge, and/or financial constraints) give her a decent chance of beating her ED? It is distressing to recall how often and persistently we had to fight the system—including her various treatment teams—to get faster or more aggressive action, or even communication about the treatment strategy. It has been a Herculean task.

The biggest danger, of course, is that in only a few weeks, those in the grips of this insidious disorder can find themselves in grave danger. Time is of the essence in order to prevent anorexia from completely hijacking the brain. We had so much to learn, and with the illness spiraling out of control, we didn't have the time required to accumulate the vital information that would have informed the questions we needed to ask, and the decisions we had to make early on.

We hope this book provides insight, knowledge about resources, and perhaps a bit of hope to others who find themselves where we were two years ago.

CHAPTER TWO:
WHAT IS IT AND WHAT CAUSES IT?

The most important thing to know up front is that anorexia is a complex psychiatric illness, with devastating physical consequences affecting all body systems, including the brain, heart, the bones, and all other vital organs. It has the highest mortality rate of any mental health disorder. The National Association of Anorexia Nervosa and Associated Disorders reports that 5-10% of anorexics die within 10 years; 18-20% within 20 years, and only 30-40% fully recover. The death rate is *12 times higher* than all other causes of death for 15-24-year-old females. Many die prematurely from complications directly related to their eating disorder, including suicide and heart problems.

As a psychiatric illness (not simply an excessive desire to be thin), many potential medical complications may ensue, including (but not limited to):

- Brain damage (which may or may not be restored fully even if the person can recover fully)
- Damage to the structure and function of the heart
- Low blood pressure, slowed breathing and pulse
- Electrolyte imbalances
- Amenorrhea (loss of menstrual cycle)
- Infertility
- Gastrointestinal problems (cramps, bloating, constipation, diarrhea, incontinence, acid reflux)
- Kidney infection and failure
- Liver failure

- Pancreatitis
- Osteoporosis or osteopenia
- Brittle nails, purple nail bed
- Dry and yellowish skin, bruising
- Drop in internal body temperature, causing a person to feel cold all the time
- Lethargy, sluggishness, feeling tired all the time
- Dehydration
- Hair loss and breakage
- Edema (swelling of soft tissues resulting from excess water accumulation from laxative or diuretic abuse)
- Hypo- and Hyperglycemia (low/high blood sugar)
- Hyponatremia (low sodium)
- Iron-deficient anemia
- Ketoacidosis (high level of acids build up when the body burns fat instead of sugar/carbs)
- Lanugo (growth of soft downy hair on face, back, and/or arms)
- Low platelet count
- Muscle atrophy
- Seizures
- Sleep problems

Many of these problems are reversible, if the person is able to restore nutritional status and increase weight to a healthy range. But we have also read and heard that some medical complications, at least for some patients, might not be completely reversible, such as brain structure and function, osteoporosis, and fertility.

Anorexia Nervosa – Common Characteristics

Anorexia is an **egosyntonic** illness. That is, the beliefs that underscore it and the behaviors that manifest from those beliefs are enmeshed with the needs and goals of the ego. Weight loss, the ability to exert excessive control over consumption, etc. become integral to one's sense of identity and self-worth, which is precisely why it is such a pernicious and complex illness.

In addition, it is an illness in which behavior is characterized by a state of **anosognosia**, in which the person is unable to sense or feel there is a problem or to connect the physical and psychological ailments they endure with their food restriction. This is considered to be a condition rooted in physiology, which is easily misunderstood as denial. However, denial is a psychological defense mechanism, be it conscious or subconscious.

Further, people in the grips of anorexia display **interoceptive** deficits, meaning an inability to perceive internal states such as pain, hunger, or thirst. This may be due to malfunctioning of the neurobiological circuitry in the brain or to problems with neuropeptides produced in the digestive tract, or perhaps to the brain receptor insensitivities for those neuropeptides. Different theories as to the cause of this phenomenon have been postulated, but the cause of the interoceptive deficits remains as yet unclear.

Finally, in acute stages of the illness, people suffering from anorexia are also often characterized by **alexythemia**, a state of deficiency in understanding, processing, or describing emotions.

Anorexia is a multifaceted disorder, and resistance to being treated is common in the acute phase of the illness. Indeed, the inability to grasp the physical danger one is in is a primary symptom of the illness.

How is anorexia diagnosed?

DSM IV, (the Diagnostic and Statistical Manual of Mental Disorders), published in 1994 and revised in July 2000, is the current diagnostic manual that health care providers and insurance companies use to diagnose mental disorders. (DSM V is scheduled for publication in May 2013). According to DSM IV, Anorexia Nervosa is:

1. Refusal to maintain normal body weight, leading to weight that is less than 85% of normal.
2. Intense fear of gaining weight or becoming fat, even though underweight.
3. Disturbance in the way one's body weight or shape is experienced, undue influence of body shape on self-evaluation, or denial of the seriousness of current low body weight.

4. The lack of at least 3 consecutive menstrual periods.

This provides just the barest technical description, and only describes a fraction of people with serious and dangerous eating disorders, a major problem in ensuring those with sub-clinical diagnoses get the care they need to prevent the condition from worsening and becoming chronic.

Aside from the DSM IV criteria, what does anorexia look like in person? Specifics differ for every person, of course. Some develop the problem gradually, which may make it more difficult to detect. In our case, it was sudden. We perceived that our daughter had a split personality, although psychiatrists tell us that people with a real diagnosis of split personality are entirely unaware when they slip into the different personas, and have no conscious recollection of having been on the other side. What we witnessed was more like a Jekyll-Hyde phenomenon. She became attacking, accusing, delusional, angry, and protective of her suddenly bizarre behaviors around food and in the kitchen. When she was home during those first few months on select weekends and then for a few weeks during spring vacation prior to her first admission to a residential treatment facility, she wouldn't eat a thing I had prepared; nor would she eat with us. If I was cooking, she would hover to make sure I didn't add oil or whatever it was in the moment she was compelled to object to. One time, when she hadn't eaten all day, I suggested she at least have some miso soup (long a favorite of hers); she hissed at me as if possessed, and adamantly refused that or anything, as if to spite me. Since suggesting that she eat caused her to refuse, I would purposely leave the kitchen in the hope that she'd at least try to fix herself something on her own. It was risking a lose-lose proposition, but there was no way she'd eat if I offered her anything; we just hoped there'd be a chance her hunger would be strong enough to cause her to make a compromise with whatever inside her was refusing to allow her to eat, on her own. This was torture for us. It was the same with buying groceries. If I bought it, she wouldn't eat it, even if I bought the few limited things she was allowing herself. In her mind, perhaps she felt I was controlling her, or giving in to what I bought meant she was losing whatever battle her eating disordered thoughts made her think she was waging against me. But then *she* wouldn't buy anything, either, and then in the kitchen she'd rant loudly about how there wasn't anything in the kitchen she could eat! She eliminated whole groups of foods she used to like, as if to punish herself (although we had no idea *why*): pastas, carbs, desserts, meats, cheese, eggs. The few times she was home, she'd eat part of an apple, a few bites of oatmeal, a granola bar, maybe some cabbage.

In addition to not accepting any offers to get her things she might eat, she started giving back to me, in what seemed a deeply spiteful manner, any non-food item I had given her: a cushion for her chair, any of the items I'd gotten her for room at school. I was crushed. I had looked so forward to getting her things when she went away, the way I wish my mom had done for me. Devastated by this turn of events, I had no answer for how I, her biggest advocate, had abruptly become Enemy #1.

We read many books (many of which were published before the advances in technology that enabled brain imagining and gene research) that hypothesize familial relationships as being the culprit. The mother, in these outdated and baseless hypotheses, is too enmeshed, too controlling, or—quite the opposite—a "refrigerator mom;" the father is emotionally distant. We now know that people who become victims of anorexia come from all family types. Families are not to blame. There simply is no evidence to support that claim.

Anorexia is often misconstrued as a means used to gain control in one's life, and some people—i.e., both treatment professionals and well-meaning friends or acquaintances—assumed that her extreme measures to gain control were directed at us, as if this was simply her way of rebelling. The implication was that we must have been oppressive control-freaks as parents. To say the least, we were devastated to feel so misconstrued. We had done everything in our power to NOT be controlling parents: we supported both daughters in taking up activities that were different from our own, and were happy that they did not feel the need to compete with our competencies. We didn't have to impose curfews, for instance, because we made our expectations clear, negotiated a time we could all agree to, and they almost always complied. We encouraged them to make their own decisions, even when they tried to defer to us, so they could practice making decisions for themselves in a way we knew they would need to do in order to succeed on their own. We feel we did most things right in terms of strengthening their wings so that when they left the nest, they would be strong enough to soar.

So, how on earth can a child, who comes from a close-knit family—where the kids know they are their parents' absolute first priority, where direct and healthy ways of communicating have been encouraged, and where all parenting decisions have been aimed at producing healthy adolescents—and who was at a perfectly normal weight for her height, end up in a situation where she'd lost her grip on reality, had become the devil incarnate in her relations with us, and above all, who was starving herself, quite possibly to death?

From all the reading we've done, we know there is no single cause for eating disorders. Certainly concerns about weight and body shape play a role, fueled by media portrayals of a standard of beauty unobtainable by the vast majority of girls. The ideal size of models has decreased from size 14 to size zero or 2. Society is obsessed with the pursuit of thinness, and thinness has come to symbolize values such as sexiness, strength, discipline, success, and happiness. But, while the cultural obsession with thinness is a factor that shouldn't be overlooked, it can't possibly be the only culprit when considering the development of a significantly dangerous illness. After all, millions of people diet to lose weight, yet only a small fraction of them end up with a severe psychiatric and medical condition.

What we know is that for many, anorexia *is* about control, but not necessarily directed at the parents or their external environments. It's about controlling deep and distressing internal chaos, anxieties and emotions too difficult to cope with. This may be driven by neurobiological factors, which in turn may be hard-wired in the genes. Some experts explain that dysregulation in certain chemicals, such as serotonin and norepinephrine, which are associated with feeding, reward and well-being, may drive those afflicted to starve, as malnutrition lowers serotonin levels and hence decreases anxiety. Over the past decade, it has become clear that genetics contribute significantly to the development of eating disorders. No single gene is believed to be responsible; rather, it is likely that many genes code for personality traits as well as the complex neural circuitry associated with food—in other words, there is a genetic underpinning to the biological processes that occur within the brain. A more in-depth explanation of this will follow shortly, but at this point, it is important to note that there is also a complex relationship between genetic predisposition and environmental factors.

It also is important to note that just because one might have a genetic predisposition toward an illness, it doesn't necessarily mean that that disposition will manifest in illness. The gene loads the gun, and environmental factors pull the trigger. This is something we have heard all along – in parent support groups, from treatment professions, at conferences, in the literature. This is a key concept to grasp, and which underscores the need for prevention programs since there's no way to know who has the genetic predisposition until a person succumbs to the illness.

Yet there is more to the story: Once starvation sets in, the malnutrition itself causes profound physiological changes in brain function, both structurally and functionally, and these changes affect thoughts, beliefs, and actions.

Some people suggest that almost everyone who becomes anorexic starts out by dieting. Surely, in a thin-obsessed culture, the pressure to be thin can be considered an environmental toxin. It's a problem when 81% of 10-year olds feel they are too fat and should diet, when 54% of women would rather be hit by a truck than be fat (from Ophelia's Place brochure), and when $60 billion is spent annually in the U.S. alone on the diet (or perhaps more accurately called the "weight cycling") industry—even though 95% of all dieters regain their lost weight in 1-5 years.

Surely, body dissatisfaction is an established risk factor for eating disorders, and this needs to be given due consideration. Yet we have also met people who have struggled with anorexia who say that the desire to be thin was never a factor in the equation. We know of one girl who had the flu, at age 11, but even after recovering she continued losing weight; she struggled with anorexia for nine years before dying at age 20. One uncovers many such stories at ED parent support groups. But prominent therapists explain that even in such cases, the desire to lose weight and associated body image issues leads to a dieting mindset and does become part of the dynamic for even rarer cases in which the anorexia didn't stem originally from the desire to find happiness through an attempt at weight loss. In short: It isn't always an obsession with thinness that triggers anorexia, but many argue it almost invariably enters the equation.

Even if not starting from a desire to be thin, not eating has disastrous consequences in the brain, especially dangerous in those susceptible genetically and otherwise, toward developing anorexia.

One well-known study demonstrated the effects of extreme dietary restriction: the Minnesota Starvation Experiment, which was conducted over the course of a year (1944-45). This study was designed, in part, to determine the physical and psychological effects of severe and prolonged dietary restriction so that the scientific results could guide the Allied relief assistance to famine victims in Europe and Asia at the end of World War II. Thirty-six normal-weight, healthy men were recruited for the experiment. For the first 12 weeks, they were given a diet of approximately 3200 calories to maintain their normal body weight, to establish a baseline. For the next 24 weeks, their caloric intake was reduced by approximately half, with the goal of inducing a 25% weight loss. The last phase was divided into two parts: a restricted and then unrestricted restoration phase.

The results of this experiment showed an astonishing similarity to the effects of starvation in those with anorexia, both physically and psychologically. Psychologically, they experienced severe emotional distress, hysteria, depression, a preoccupation with food during the starvation and rehabilitation phase, social withdrawal, isolation, et al. One person even amputated three of his fingers with an axe! The results of the study underscore the belief that severe malnutrition has profound social and psychological impact, and that recovery depends on physical re-nourishment as well as psychological treatment.

Anorexia is considered a biopsychosocial illness. Some people seem to be genetically hard-wired, with a vulnerability of risk for eating disorders, both with regard to biological and neurological dysregulations in the brain, as well as with regard to the temperamental traits and cognitive styles inherent in the afflicted individual. It is thus an amalgam of genetics, neurobiological factors and environmental stressors that—under certain circumstances—can become a toxic stew, one might say.

Twin and family studies have recently shown that anorexia is eight times more common in people who have relatives with the disorder. Twins also have a tendency to share particular eating disorders (anorexia nervosa, bulimia nervosa, and obesity). Researchers have identified specific chromosomes that may be associated with bulimia and anorexia. According to Wade Berrettini, MD, PhD, investigators have identified a likely susceptibility gene for AN located at chromosome 1p34. However, "a single susceptibility gene is neither necessary nor sufficient for the development of AN," he said, adding that an affected person must inherit several susceptibility genes, each of which produces a small increase in risk for the disorder. Even then, the appropriate environmental influences must also be present."

UC San Diego's Dr. Walter Kaye, a leader in brain imaging and research on eating disorders, asserts that there are some 43 genes involved in the regulation of eating behavior, motivation and rewards, and studies show consistent associations identified with several brain chemicals and neurotransmitters, including serotonin, dopamine, BNRF, and AgRP. It is believed that a dysregulation in serotonin, which is linked to anxiety, mood, and impulse control, may create vulnerability for the expression of symptoms and may contribute to the etiology of eating disorders. It turns out that starvation or prolonged malnutrition may actually cause a malfunction in the neurotransmitters in the brain of those with eating disorders: it is believed to actually decrease the serotonin in the brain, producing the calming effect desperately sought after in those experiencing anxiety.

In addition to serotonin, two other neurotransmitters regulate stress, mood and appetite, and may play a role in the development of eating disorders. Imbalances in norepinephrine, which is a stress hormone, and dopamine, which is involved in reward-seeking behavior, may explain in part why those with anorexia do not experience a sense of pleasure from food and other typical comforts.

Currently, the mechanism for how an inherited susceptibility to eating disorders might work is not completely understood. One possibility is that temperament—the biological aspect of an individual's personality that is present at birth and forms the basis for adult personality—may play a factor. Presently, it's unclear whether brain dysfunctions noted in those with anorexia cause the disorder, or whether starvation itself causes brain changes that perpetuate self-starvation.

Could it be that our daughter's increasing depression and anxieties, which escalated through her high school years, reached a critical mass when she went off to college, exacerbated by a desire to be as skinny as her best friend, which caused her to diet and to not feel like eating (lack of appetite is common with depression)? Did this in turn create a chemical reaction in her brain that allowed her to feel in control of her unspoken and massive anxieties, setting a vicious cycle in motion? Could she quell her internal turmoil while simultaneously conquering what so many others find difficult to manage, i.e., sustained weight loss?

After several months of being in the trenches with this illness, it dawned on us that our daughter might also have a constitution that is sensitive to not eating. I love to cook, and home-cooked family meals are a big thing at our house; we often have friends over for meals, so there aren't many occasions for people to skip meals when food plays such a central role in our life.

We can recall an instance when she was in 1st grade that now stands out eerily, and we now wonder whether it may have been a precursor to her anorexia. (Little did we know then!) The transition from kindergarten to 1st grade was a big one for her, though we didn't really know why. Her moods became suddenly quite erratic, and we learned that she wasn't eating snack during recess. In addition, she often came home with her lunch uneaten. We suspected that her moods were caused by not eating; we figured it was a blood sugar problem. We started experimenting with nutritional milkshakes from the health food store—the 40-30-30 blends—in her favorite flavors. Offered to her at school pick-up time along with an explanation that they were good for her and would make her feel better, she almost always refused them. (A power-control issue at age 6?!?) However, left in the cup holder of our van without comment, and unprompted, she'd usually drink them on the way home. On the days she drank those nutritional shakes, her moods were fairly even. But when she wouldn't or didn't eat, God help us!

Another occasion stands out: I had a parent meeting to go to one evening. She hadn't eaten, even after she got home from school. As I left, I cautioned my husband to make sure she ate dinner. He chose not to do so, later explaining that she hadn't said she was hungry! By the time I got home, I encountered a horrible situation. He had put her in the bath, and some now-forgotten dispute had triggered an angry outbreak, whereupon she lashed out and hit him in the face! I found him utterly devastated. I knew instinctively it had been due to a lack of food. Luckily, this issue seemed to resolve itself in time, and there were no more battles about food or control until high school, when I harped on the girls regarding the need to eat a good breakfast before they went to school, an issue that comes up often with teenage girls. It's not only important to start out the day with good nutrition, but not doing so also sets people up for uncontrolled binging when they get home from school half starved, which of course leads to feelings of remorse and self-hatred. No amount of rational discussion seemed to get through to them. So, to help them avoid binging on snack foods in the afternoon between school and sports practice, I made a point of having dinner prepared and left on the stove, ready for them to have in the late afternoon – this was, at least ensuring that when they ate, they were eating nutritious and balanced food!

The episode of her mood swings in first grade still haunts us: Was her sensitivity to not eating part of a vulnerability that led her to anorexia in late adolescence? Had the eating disorder made an unrecognized debut in her as a child, only to lie dormant until the stresses of late adolescence provoked its eruption?

If one were to try to grasp how anorexia develops, purely from a psychological level, this is how we have often heard it described: First, there's generalized anxiety, lack of self-esteem (in spite of incredible capability and achievement, objectively speaking), and a state of agitation caused by any number of personal challenges. In this state, many pursue dieting to gain control of those bad feelings – to feel a little better, somehow. (This is where the cultural obsession with dieting, weight loss and thinness comes in.) At this point, they lose a little weight, and people notice, saying things: "Wow, you look great! How'd you do that?" These external rewards provide a sense of achievement, and hunger pangs begin to signal a feeling of success. At some point – and it is not clear how or when – the initial goal of dropping some weight is replaced by a continuing compulsion to lose. The ability to do what most people can't (i.e., keep losing weight) provides self-gratification, and before long the compulsion drowns out all other considerations. Weight loss has now become the salve for anxiety. It becomes entwined with a sense of identity. It becomes who they are, and what they feel good at. Family or friends (or even unwitting strangers!) at this point may begin to express concern, withdraw from, or criticize someone for being too thin, but by this time, given the egosyntonic effects of this illness, the anorexia causes both an angry defiance, a misplaced sense of personal power, and a disengagement from their social milieu, contributing to the isolation that already sets in as a result of trying to avoid the many social settings that involve eating. Anorexia is an extremely isolating illness, and in this isolation, anorexia becomes a tyrannical voice in the head of someone trying to establish their sense of identity, as dangerously misguided as that is.

The defiance and all-consuming vigilance with weight—and with food and how not to eat it—having taken over, not only causes isolation but also a loss of humor. At this stage, their special thinness becomes entwined with their newfound assertiveness. The stage is set for anorexia to *become their identity*, and efforts by others to re-feed them are experienced as attempts to rob them of their sense of self. We are not sure if this is the exact progression of our daughter's illness, but as our daughter said, more than once in the throes of her anorexia, "This is just the way I am; deal with it."

What of the inborn inclinations, temperament and cognitive style so common to those who develop anorexia? Brain studies have shown a clear tendency for those who struggle with anorexia to be anxiety prone; they push themselves hard; they are highly self-critical; and they are perfectionists: Nothing is ever good enough. (There's an obsessive nature to that perfectionism, too, which is a dangerous state of mind because perfection is inherently unattainable.) They are typically risk-averse, tend toward negative thought patterns, and are often introverted. They have a rigid cognitive style, i.e., they are rule bound, regard life internally and externally in black-and-white terms; and have difficulty in set shifting (demonstrating flexibility in the face of changing rules, parameters or reinforcements). They are known to have problems with central coherence, which in laymen's terms means they can't see or appreciate the forest because they're obsessing about the details of the trees. Research suggests that some or all of those traits are at least partially driven by genetics.

Individuals with anorexia and bulimia tend to be quite competitive, and are driven to succeed. They often compare their appearance and accomplishments against unrealistic standards and find themselves lacking. Their judgments involve culturally derived or peer-sanctioned standards rather than inner-conceived expectations; i.e., people with eating disorders are primarily concerned about what others think, rather than what they think of themselves. Other people with eating disorders, such as athletes, tend to judge themselves against internally derived standards, and get upset when they fail to live up to their own ideals, expectations and goals, regardless of how unrealistic those may be.

Regardless of which set of standards are used, perfectionists strive to meet the highest standard of performance possible. They easily find themselves in a self-defeating cycle of fear and dissatisfaction when they fail to meet their expectations and goals. This sense of unmet goals becomes the fuel and the motivation that perpetuates a renewed drive toward thinness, perfection, and the need for control. Hence, the vicious cycle of dysfunctional eating behaviors that constitute eating disorders.

We read all that and were dumbstruck: How could they know our daughter so well? They had described her to a T. And how could we, who know her so well, not have a clue that all that might manifest in self-starvation; might render her unable to sense the danger of malnutrition; might result in a delusional state of mind such that she could not attribute her exhaustion, perpetually being cold (even in warm weather), thinning hair or blue nail beds to malnourishment. It is also conceivable that she *did* make those connections but took perverted pride in having been strong enough to take the dieting to such an extreme. It is also conceivable that she made those connections but felt powerless to fight the forces (a voice? fear? negative thoughts?) that were causing her to restrict.

We often hear professionals describe the phenomenon of eating disorders described as a situation in which genetics load the gun and the environment pulls the trigger. Another way to describe it is to imagine a flask in a chemistry experiment.

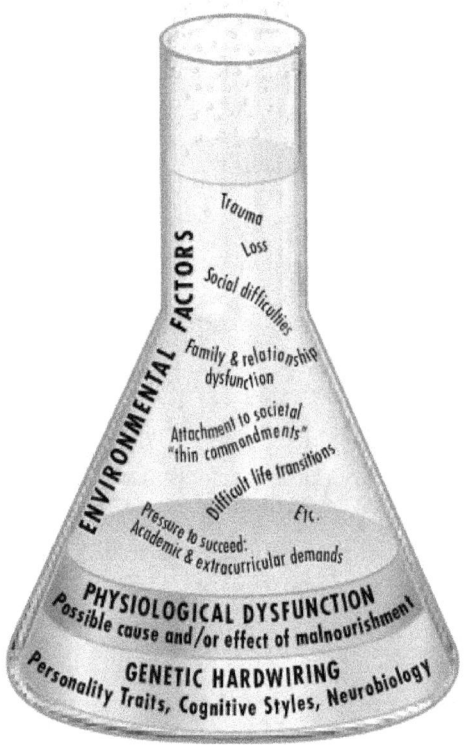

The flask is a finite size. Once it becomes full, it explodes into an eating disorder. Let's say that the value, the critical mass, as it were, after which an ED is born – when the flask is full - is a value of 100. Each eating disorder flask has as its substrate genetic predispositions (for common personality traits, cognitive styles, and neurobiological dysregulations). This is a given. In addition, physiological dysfunctions in the brain that either contribute to the development of, or are known to exacerbate or are caused by severe malnourishment or semi-starvation, are part of the picture. These include but are not limited to abnormal levels of serotonin, dopamine, and other chemicals that cause maladaptive synapses in the brain of those suffering, such that they don't respond in the same way to hunger or satiety, etc. (Dr. Walter Kaye, from UC San Diego, addresses these phenomena in his research, should you care to delve further on this topic.)

In effect, flasks without a genetic hardwiring substrate won't result in an eating disorder, and those which don't reach a critical mass, based on all contributing factors, won't develop into a full-fledged eating disorder, but may remain in the gray area of subclinical eating disorders or disordered eating. Only those flasks in which the added environmental factors are great enough will. These environmental components could include: excessive pressure to succeed academically and in extra-curricular activities; an attachment to our society's obsession with the "thin ideal;" difficult social or family relationship problems; life transitions; loss, trauma, or abuse; and/or an inability to express emotions. This list could contain a multitude of other external factors, any or all of which combined with an internal hard-wired disposition toward the drive for perfection (which being unattainable leads to a sense of low self-worth, depression, and anxiety) are factors that combine to some degree toward the development of an eating disorder.

No single individual who develops an eating disorder will struggle with the same set of environmental problems, nor will each issue carry the same weight. However, when the value (of the combination of the particular environmental factors mixed with the genetic underpinnings of the illness) reaches the top of the flask, it's a toxic brew, the lid of the flask bursts, and illness ensues.

CHAPTER THREE:
LEVELS OF CARE

In order to fully understand the different levels of treatment of anorexia, it is helpful to briefly review the basics of this disorder:

Anorexia nervosa (AN) is a psychiatric disorder with severe physiologic consequences, characterized by the inability or refusal to maintain a minimally normal weight. Patients have a profoundly disturbed body image as well as an intense fear of weight gain despite being moderately to severely underweight, defined as below 85% of ideal body weight. Amenorrhea, or loss of menstruation (for at least three cycles), in girls who have already started their periods, is also included in the description used in the *Diagnostic and Statistical Manual of Mental Disorders IV (DSM-IV)*, details of which are included in the next chapter.

Anorexia nervosa may be divided into two subtypes: (1) restricting, in which severe limitation of food intake is the primary means to weight loss, and (2) binge-eating/purging type, in which there are periods of food intake that are compensated by self-induced vomiting, laxative or diuretic abuse, and/or excessive exercise.

Formal recommendations have been made to remove the amenorrhea criterion and the subtype distinctions from the criteria for anorexia nervosa in the upcoming *DSM-V*. In addition, it has been suggested that *DSM-V* be expanded to include sub-threshold eating disorders that don't fit the specific criteria listed, as there are many people struggling with severe disorders that don't meet each criteria, and they are often just as serious and life-threatening as those that fit all criteria. Without this expansion of the category, these victims will continue to be denied the treatment they desperately need.

With eating disorders being psychiatric illnesses that cause both profound and dangerous changes in the body, all of which directly relate to the amount of food consumed, it stands to reason that patients with anorexia and other eating disorders should be seen and treated by professionals who have demonstrable expertise in each of these areas. In addition, the clinicians should work as a team so that the treatment plan can be developed with input regarding all components of the illness.

Physicians need to be involved to regularly monitor weight, vitals (blood pressure, heart rate, etc.) hormone levels, and electrolyte levels, etc. (This is not, however, a comprehensive list).

Nutritionists need to help patients establish and monitor food plans, and support them in overcoming their diminished ability to feed themselves —a particularly difficult task because it requires the establishment of trust to overpower the "voice" directing an eating disordered client to do the opposite of what the nutritionist is there do to do.

Therapists can assist by guiding the client to deeper insights and providing emotional assistance (which comes in many forms). This will be discussed in the following chapter.

Psychiatrists may need to get involved to establish whether there are dual diagnoses involved, as well as whether and when pharmacology can help relieve symptoms. Unfortunately, there is no pill that cures anorexia. Most medications, it turns out, have only limited success in combatting the associated depression, anxiety, obsessive-compulsive and psychotic elements of the disease. Some medications won't be effective at all in underweight patients. Apparently, SSRIs such as Prozac and the like, have proven particularly ineffective with anorexic patients in the acute phase of the disease (i.e., when significantly underweight), and some of the newer antipsychotic medications, some of which have shown some limited success in reducing some symptoms, are not tolerated well due to side effects patients don't like. It is also very difficult to find comprehensive research studies because the drop-out rate in this population is known to be extremely high.

Together, the team must develop (and keep refining) a plan, monitor the patient, and communicate with each other on their observations week to week. This coordination does not necessarily happen well in an outpatient setting, as we found out; this can also be quite problematic, as we will describe in the next chapter.

Initially, we had no idea what different kinds of care are out there, much less that there are established levels of care. Below are three places you can find information that explains the criteria used to establish which level of care is appropriate.

- The American Psychiatric Association (APA) Practice Guidelines: Treatment of Patients With Eating Disorders, Third Edition. If you go to this site, scroll down to Table 8. http://psychiatryonline.org/content.aspx?bookid=28&sectionid=1671334#138660.

- The National Eating Disorder Association (NEDA) publishes toolkits for parents, educators and athletic coaches. Visit the "NEDA Toolkit for Parents" site to find this, among other useful pieces of information: that explains the criteria used for establishing which level of care is appropriate. http://www.nationaleatingdisorders.org/uploads/file/toolkits/NEDA-TKP-B04-TreatmentSettingsAndCare.pdf.

- Additionally, attorney warrior Lisa Kantor, who fights insurance companies on behalf of eating disorder clients and their families, has similar information on her website: http://www.kantorlaw.net/Areas_of_Practice/Eating_Disorders/Conferences/2011_IAEDP_Materials.aspx.

Generally speaking, the level of care is determined by the acuteness and severity of the medical, emotional and behavioral issues involved in the illness. The intensity and duration of treatment at any given treatment level will depend on many factors, unfortunately including insurance coverage.

Treatment professionals will likely recommend the appropriate level of care, but this is not necessarily the case, as some providers of care who are not expert or experienced may not know. As parents, it is important to know that there are five levels of treatment. In addition, patients do not necessarily start at Level 1 and progress up through the levels (nor do the levels follow any prescribed order); nor do they necessarily go down a level as symptoms improve. We found it helpful to research the options at each level in our geographic area ahead of time so that we could be informed participants when treatment options were discussed.

The five levels of care are:

> Level 1: Outpatient Care.
>
> Level 2: Intensive Outpatient Care (IOP).
>
> Level 3. Partial Hospitalization Program (PHP), also known as "Day Treatment"
>
> Level 4: Residential Treatment
>
> Level 5. Inpatient Hospitalization

Level 1: Outpatient Care

Outpatient care entails weekly (or some other regularly scheduled) appointments with a physician, a nutritionist, and a therapist, and possibly also a psychiatrist. In general, Level 1 care is indicated when a patient is medically stable, is generally at least about 85% of healthy body weight, has fair-to-good motivation, seems to be self-sufficient with regard to the level of structure needed for eating or gaining weight, and can manage the compulsion to over-exercise (if that is part of the disorder's presentation). It is important to note that you may be responsible for finding each of the various treatment providers at this level of care. There may be some "IOP" facilities that offer access to a team of physicians, nutritionists and therapists, but in many cases, people have to find providers on their own. It is important to find a physician (or therapist or registered dietician) who has experience with and can pull together a team willing to communicate with each other and with you in order to provide proper care based each of their regular assessments.

Level 2: Intensive Outpatient Care (IOP)

Intensive outpatient care is offered in a variety of settings, and what we found is that program offerings are not standardized. Some facilities offer a specific schedule of 3-4 hours per day, including a group lunch (or dinner) and snack with specific therapy groups (which may include discussions on "food and feelings," art therapy, or process groups, or more structured and didactic cognitive behavior or dialectical behavior groups). Others, such as the only IOP facility in our daughter's college town, offer a meeting with the nutritionist, a meeting with a therapist (either on staff, or out in the community) and several evening groups, but no formal supported meal program! (We had to request meal support; the most they would commit to was one meal per week.) Some IOPs told us they would not accept patients who are not motivated to participate in their recovery. This is particularly problematic when dealing with patients struggling with an egosyntonic illness, and who may go in and out of different levels of motivation.

Intensive outpatient treatment (IOP) is indicated when patients are medically stable, are psychiatrically stable, don't need daily medical monitoring, and whose symptoms are under sufficient enough control that they can function in social, education, and vocational settings. While some patients may enter treatment at this level, others may move to this level if progress isn't being made, or motivation to recover is lacking in an outpatient (Level I) setting. However, IOP is often used as a step-down setting from a higher level of care. They may step down from a PHP or residential setting, or they may even enter this setting upon discharge from an inpatient hospital setting. For example, utilizing IOP after PHP may be necessary has a step toward independent living, after learning better survival tools in a residential setting; similarly, it may be used after medical stabilization has been achieved after being discharged from a hospital in order to learn tools that can't be learned in short hospital stays.

Level 3: Partial Hospitalization Program (PHP)

PHP programs are full-day programs that clients attend 4-6 days per week. These days usually last 7-8 hours, and often include two main meals and one or two snacks per day, as well as weekly individual therapy appointments, and a variety of mandatory group meetings. Some facilities offer individual family psychotherapy as an essential component; others don't. Unfortunately, we chose a facility for our daughter that said individual family psychotherapy as an integral component, but when it was too late (i.e., she was already well into the program), we discovered that wasn't true.

PHPs are offered in a variety of settings, including some IOPs, inpatient hospital programs, and residential treatment facilities, although this latter venue would offer it only to patients who have just completed a residential treatment course at that facility, as a "step-down" program.

PHPs are not utilized only as a step-down from residential treatment. The treatment team in an outpatient or IOP setting may feel the patient can manage in a PHP instead of a residential facility; it may be that PHP is selected when there are no spaces available in the residential facility at the time treatment is required, so PHP is the next best level of care available; it may be that the patient will agree to participate in a PHP but not in residential, even if residential care is indicated and available; this may be a level higher than before and better than staying put; or it may be that insurance refuses to cover the costs of residential care. Residential care ranges from $1000-$1300 *per day*—obviously, a significant amount if parents must pay out-of-pocket. Residential stays often last from one to several months in duration: A three-month stay could cost $100,000.

PHP-level care is indicated when the patient is medically stable but whose motivation is unstable or lacking; when body weight is still well below normal; and/or when the patient is preoccupied with intrusive, repetitive thoughts for more than a few hours per day.

Level 4: Residential Treatment Centers

Residential treatment centers are mostly stand-alone facilities, and there are some 75 such facilities in the U.S. (according to the New York Times, October 15, 2011). There are residential facilities for adolescents (age 10-18 or 19), some for adults (18 and older), even a few for men and boys. There are apparently facilities in England for pre-pubescent children struggling with anorexia and other eating disorders.

Each residential facility has its own rules. Those for adults are not locked facilities. If the going gets rough, patients can leave of their own accord. And the going does get tough. We've heard many stories of patients who left prematurely, against the advice of the treatment teams.

Residential treatment is indicated in instances when there is an acute weight decline (even if not to below 85% of body weight); motivation is poor; and when there is preoccupation with intrusive, repetitive thoughts throughout the day. It is also indicated when there is resistance to treatment at other levels or when compliance and cooperation may occur only in a highly structured environment. At the residential level, supervision during and after all meals is necessary for a time, in order to prevent restriction or the binge/purge cycle, and for those with exercise addiction, full-time assistance is needed to help break the exercise habit. Residential treatment facilities provide structured schedules, including regular visits with the doctor, nurse, and nutritionist; a therapist for individual sessions several times a week; and mandatory participation in group discussions.

Each facility operates under varying beliefs. Some focus on nutritional and weight restoration before the client is expected to fully participate in the various psychological therapies. Others are less concerned with participation until enough time has gone by to allow the brain to recalibrate, which some feel is required for a person with anorexia to be able to think rationally enough to make use of the sessions. Some believe in the value of a fast-paced weight gain; others feel a gradual strategy is more sustainable. Some hold that a step-down to a PHP program is essential to successful treatment; others don't recommend this (or at least don't insist on it). Some discharge a client as soon as "sufficient" weight gain has been achieved; others feel it is necessary for a client to maintain the weight gained for a time before discharge in order to allow the psyche to catch up with their new body, this in the belief that it will reduce the chance that the gained weight won't be lost as soon as the client leaves the facility. It may be important to determine the philosophy of the treatment team before you commit to sending your child there. Oftentimes, physicians or other professionals on the team are not well acquainted with the particular philosophies of the residential facilities they refer to, so the more information you have, the better informed your choice will be.

Our experience suggests that stepping down from a residential treatment facility to a day treatment program provides essential support in transitioning back into normal life, especially if that life means a return to one or more of the stressors that were problematic prior to entering residential treatment. It's one thing to eat in a setting where everyone at the table is similarly struggling, and in which not eating will result in being fed supplements or being hospitalized. It's quite another to apply the skills learned in residential setting back in one's home environment, or on their own, when the scaffolding of care is suddenly no longer available. In a residential setting, eating-disordered thoughts and impulses increasingly take back seat out of necessity. In the real world, those struggling with food, weight, body size and shape have to make multitudes of food-related decisions each day on their own, be it purchasing groceries, cooking, eating with family and friends (or alone), going to restaurants, being in the company of others who they might envy for their thinness, or quite often, handling the internal battle that ensues when people comment on how they look. These and many other issues that cause anxiety can trigger anorexic behaviors.

A step-down to PHP and IOP settings provide more support for taking on these challenges. Consider that in residential, three snacks and three meals are consumed each day in a supported environment. That means 42 situations per week where clients are directly confronting food fears or eating difficulties, yet have therapists on hand to help them cope *in the moment*. In PHP, if they are only eating two meals and one snack daily, they are already managing 50% of their meals on their own. It affords plenty of opportunity to restrict enough to cause weight loss following residential treatment even if they eat all meals provided in a PHP setting. In other words, if they feel they are eating too much during their meals in PHP treatment, they might be hard pressed to make and eat, say, a complete breakfast (consisting, perhaps, of a couple fried eggs, a couple pieces of buttered toast, sausage, a glass of milk and a fruit) on their own, during the rest of the meals throughout the week that are not supervised. You can see, then, that even PHP is chancy enough following residential treatment. Skipping a step-down program and going to even an IOP, with fewer supported meals, or outpatient care, with no supported meals, is hugely risky. With relapse rates for those leaving residential treatment so high, why skip this step?

Level 5: Inpatient Hospitalization

Hospitalization is generally short-term measure when a patient is in medical
danger and needs to be monitored and stabilized. It could be due to
bradycardia (slow heart rate) or other cardiac dysrhythmias, severe electrolyte
(potassium, sodium, or phosphorous) abnormalities, altered mental status or
suicidality, extremely low body weight (usually less than 75%), or failure of
outpatient treatment. Patients are often discharged as soon as they meet the
minimum weight and other requirements. Average length of stays have
shortened over time, with some hospitals saying their average is somewhere
between one and two weeks. Insurance companies, as well, will often not
cover hospital stays once a patient is stabilized. While one might hope that
the patient can stay in a hospital longer, many treatment professionals prefer
that the hospital stay be as short as possible so the patient can receive the
intensive and focused treatment that hospitals are not designed to provide.

We suggest calling your local hospitals (or those near where your child lives)
to find out which ones offer units dedicated to eating disorders. Ask the
physician on your treatment team which hospital he or she would admit your
child to, if it were to become necessary. If you passively allow the doctor to
make that choice, your child may be admitted to a hospital without an eating
disorder unit. In this case, they will be placed in a general unit or a psychiatric
unit, and it's not likely there will be staff qualified to manage eating
disordered patients (i.e., who understand the complexities of the illness,
including the tricks that patients use to avoid food intake). Even if the closest
hospital with a dedicated eating disorders unit is some distance away, tell the
doctor this is your preference in case hospitalization becomes necessary.
Obtain the doctor's agreement and cooperation early on, so that you aren't
scrambling when time is short and emotions are high; you may also need to
look into potential insurance complications for coverage at a hospital out of
your immediate geographic area.

In our daughter's college town, there were only two hospitals, neither of
which had the capacity to manage eating disordered patients, nor did they
have the staff who understood the illness or the behaviors that need to be
monitored. In one hospital, she would have been on a general floor; in the
other she would have been admitted to the psychiatric unit. We were worried

that if her health continued to deteriorate, she wouldn't be able to get home in time to be admitted to the hospital in our town that does have an eating disorder unit. When we asked the college doctor which hospital she would refer our daughter to, we were floored to learn that she wasn't sure, herself! We were glad we had done the research ourselves.

Here is a sampling of hospitals that have dedicated eating disorder units:

- El Camino Hospital, in Mountain View, California, which houses Stanford University's Lucile Packard Children's Hospital's Eating Disorder Unit

  - Alta Bates Medical Center, in Berkeley, California, which houses the Center for Anorexia and Bulimia (offering inpatient and outpatient programs)

  - Children's Hospital in Denver, Colorado (offering inpatient as well as a PHP/IOP program). The philosophy in this program is that family is the most important and effective component of successful intervention. At least one parent is required to attend on a daily basis for the entire period of care. The model includes PSN (parent supported nutrition) in which the parent prepares and provides the meals; the program utilizes family therapy as well as individual therapy. This is a unique program in this country.

These are but three examples of hospitals with dedicated eating disorder units, to give an idea of the different types and locations. As noted above, we strongly encourage *early* investigation into hospitals and other resources, whenever possible; you will be at a distinct disadvantage if you wait until the need for services is imminent.

PART TWO: WHAT ARE THE MOST IMPORTANT THINGS TO KNOW AT THE OUTSET?

CHAPTER FOUR: THE DIVIDE BETWEEN RESEARCH AND TREATMENT, AND IT'S IMPLICATIONS

Perhaps the most important thing to understand is that there is often a significant divide between research and treatment; not knowing this can be hugely problematic when you are trying to get help for your child.

As has been stated previously, upon being confronted with this illness, we read everything we could get our hands on; we sent queries to professionals wherever we could find them; and we started attending parent support groups. We did all that (and more) because we felt we had no choice: Our daughter's life depended on it. But it took a while to get a handle on all the literature that exists in the field, to distinguish (and make sense of) what is current and what is "old school" thinking, to find out which theories—and their corresponding treatments—are based on *assumptions* regarding the causes of the illness, rather than on the empirical data gathered from more recent brain and genetic studies. Simply put (and not surprisingly): Treatment methodologies corresponding to the most current research have a much higher rate of effectiveness.

What we learned came too late, because our ability to absorb the material couldn't outpace the speed with which this disorder spiraled out of control in our daughter. By the time we figured that out, she was firmly in the hands of her first treatment team, and she would not have tolerated our stepping in to change her team to other professionals who we perceived were more on top of the latest research. Had we understood the nature of the divide between research and treatment, we would have known better than to hand her off to care providers steeped in the "old school" approach to the disorder.

Separately, we know now that her college town has a dearth of specialists of either the "old" or "new" schools of thought. Had we known that, we probably would not have chosen for her to return at the beginning of this roller coaster ride, so that she could have received treatment immediately from those nearby who (we now understand) are involved in cutting-edge research and treatment. Knowing that might have prevented her from wallowing in this quagmire; it could have shaved precious time off of the two years that followed.

Another reason we couldn't make changes in our approach once the ball was rolling is that in the early stages of her illness, she fiercely maintained we didn't know what we were talking about; she was also 18 and desperately trying to achieve independence and autonomy, and we had to be very careful not to feed into her perception (which could fuel the entrenchment of this disorder) that we were trying to control her. To make matters worse, her team also believed that our involvement was an encroachment on our daughter's autonomy and would interfere with her recovery. They seemed to infer that our desperate, no-holds-barred response to this unforeseen intruder in our lives must be indicative of how we raised her, and extrapolated from this that our "overbearing" ways must have been at least part of the *cause* of her illness.

It is worth considering why some professionals who treat patients with anorexia are not aware of the latest data. The sheer complexity of eating disorders may be one factor in dissuading them from keeping up with the latest findings. But the fact that the study and understanding of eating disorders is challenging and/or may be regarded as a relatively "new" science is no excuse; indeed, is it not all the more reason to keep learning and to make use of the latest developments?

Even if professionals are aware of the latest research, they may resist incorporating it into treatment plans. Perhaps this is due to a natural tendency to keep using whatever approach they were taught or have utilized in developing their practices; in some cases we perceived a tenacious hold on what was comfortable and known to them, regardless of the results. If a therapist ascribes to the common but outdated view, for example, that eating disorders are primarily emotion-based responses to internal states and external factors and that only 40% or less can recover, this is a dangerously limited—and self-limiting—belief system.

Along the way, we also experienced considerable professional arrogance. We were told that *they were the experts because they'd been immersed in the field for so long*, and that we should just back off and let them do their jobs. That was problematic, because we needed to understand the rationale for their actions (and inactions), not only as a way to understand what they were doing but to find out whether they *knew* what they were doing. Confronted with an illness for which a timely and effective treatment can mean the difference between total recovery and a lifetime of mental and physical torture punctuated by costly and lengthy stays in residential treatment, parents don't have the luxury of waiting around with blind faith that treatment providers truly understand how to combat the illness and are committed to ensuring full recovery (assuming they believe full recovery *is* possible).

If they base their treatment decisions on the assumption that only a small fraction of patients can recover, or if they believe that anorexia is simply an emotional and psychological disorder and fail to incorporate the fact that *starvation alone causes neurotransmitter malfunctions in the brain*—much of which can be reversed if re-nourishing the brain is started as early in the process as possible—then that treatment is seriously deficient (bordering on malpractice). Treatment methodologies that focus initially on psycho-education (including group or individual therapy) at the expense of nutritional restoration are allowing the illness to become more entrenched in the brain circuitry.

It was quite dismaying to find that some of our daughter's treatment providers didn't even know the names of leaders in the field, much less the nature or results of their work. To add insult to injury, we were usually brushed off when we asked questions, as if our being curious enough to want to fully understand our daughter's situation was an insult to her providers' professional integrity.

Choosing a Medical Doctor

We have heard, more than once, that medical doctors receive no more than one day of instruction on eating disorders in medical school. Whether this is precisely true or not, even physicians who have come to specialize in this field will tell you how little training they received in medical school on eating disorders.

We have heard many stories from parents distressed about their children's weight loss, bizarre eating behaviors, and personality changes—often teenagers who are either late getting their periods, or who have lost them along the way—who have taken their children to their family pediatricians (usually generalists untrained in eating disorders who will make a referral to a specialist only if they suspect a problem). These stories revolve around doctors not having found anything on lab tests (if they even go that far), and telling the parents the kids are fine, they're within normal range, and advising that the kids go home and eat more.

When a parent suspects a problem and the doctor says all is fine—this is hugely problematic because the doctor has now inadvertently colluded with the eating disorder and dismissed the parents' legitimate concerns. This makes it very difficult for the parent to provide the proper care in a timely fashion because thereafter when the parent expresses concern to the child, the child will mimic what the doctor said. We've even heard patients at various stages of recovery recount instances when they sought out care, knowing secretly that they had a severe disorder, and yet were told by doctors that there was nothing wrong with them. Unfortunately, when the eating disorder is stronger than the healthy part of their psyche (which overpowered the eating disordered thoughts enough to get them to the doctor in the first place), hearing from a doctor that nothing is wrong makes it very difficult to counter the doctor's advice, especially when their grip on reality is fragile and sporadic. These people reported that they went home defeated and further entrapped by their eating disordered thoughts and behaviors.

As a parent, it's natural to doubt your own fears when a medical authority says that all is well. Second-guessing yourself, you may choose not to pursue a second opinion. Maybe you're just being paranoid, you think. This puts parents in a tough spot, since they're dealing with an illness known to become more severe the longer it goes untended or treated ineffectually. Beliefs and behaviors become more entrenched as time goes on.

One physician—a pediatrician and respected author on eating disorders for whom we have a deep and abiding respect—said in a public lecture that she is certain she misdiagnosed many eating disorder patients in her first several years of practice as a general pediatrician, now that she has devoted her practice entirely to eating disorders for the last 15 years. One can appreciate her candor while still finding her admission frightening for what it says about the kind of care one can expect from the majority of doctors who are inadequately trained to recognize the symptoms of ED.

So how are you supposed to know if the professionals you interview have the qualifications to understand, properly diagnose, and provide treatment for these special cases? First, you can ask them what their qualifications are, and what kind of experience they have had in treating eating disordered patients. If you go to a generalist, you can insist on a referral to a specialist. Or you may want to skip the referral step and go directly to a specialist (you may have to pay out-of-pocket if your health insurance doesn't allow the direct approach to a qualified professional).

The International Association of Eating Disorders Professionals (IAEDP) is making an effort to address this problem, by providing courses that lead to certification. You can search on their website for professionals who have earned the certification and even find out what it takes to become certified. You can find specialists (physicians, nutritionists, therapists, and various treatment centers) on many other websites listed in the resource section at the back of this book.

But, at the time, we didn't know enough to ask about qualifications, experience, or knowledge. We assumed if they are "experts" in the field that they must be well versed in the latest research findings.

Choosing a Therapist

When it became clear our daughter needed help (and was refusing to seek help on her own due to her denial that anything was wrong), we searched the Internet to find a therapist in her college town with expertise and experience with eating disorder patients. 22 therapists listed themselves as experts in eating disorders, but most were on neither of our insurance panels. We were so desperate that we engaged the first one (covered by our insurance) who returned our call on that holiday weekend.

Again, what we didn't know was that we could have asked the therapist for her qualifications. Was she a member of the IAEDP? Had she received specific training and received certification through that organization? Did she frequent annual conferences put on by NEDA and other national organizations? Had she published any materials? Was she familiar with key specialists such as Drs. Treasure, Kaye, Lock, LeGrange, Fitzpatrick, et al? What books would she recommend on the topic? What was her take on the etiology of this illness? Was she familiar with the Minnesota Starvation Study and what it revealed about the psychological effects of malnutrition even when people aren't preoccupied with body image and weight loss? These are just a few of the questions we wish we'd known enough to ask.

In addition, we weren't aware of the many different therapy modalities that therapists may employ. Nor did we know that many of the different treatment modalities have yet to be studied for efficacy in comparative, long-term studies. Most importantly, we didn't understand that *the modalities employed are informed by the assumptions each provider has regarding the etiology and nature of the illness.* In retrospect, knowing this would have been key to getting appropriate care for our daughter.

We have come to understand that no specific psychotherapy approach works for every client, and that there is no consistently effective treatment for adults with anorexia nervosa. What is known is that different approaches, or a combination thereof, may work for some but not for others. It is also common knowledge that the therapeutic alliance—that is, the trust relationship between the client and provider—is a primary key to recovery. The need to trust one's therapist is tremendously magnified for people struggling with eating disorders, because heeding advice is tantamount to giving up what has become an essential part of their identity.

It may be helpful to become familiar with the types of therapies that are commonly used when treating patients with anorexia, and understand the assumptions that inform those approaches as well as the expectations that therapists have regarding chances for recovery. In the beginning, we didn't know enough to ask what type of therapy would be used, or why, and over time when we learned more about the various modalities and had questions about treatment rationale, we got very little information from the treatment teams. Once an adult child is in treatment, therapists hesitate to discuss anything with parents in order to protect patients' privacy, establish trust and develop a therapeutic alliance with clients. Patients have to feel that communication with the therapist is sacrosanct; otherwise, there is no trust, no honest communication about issues, etc. The need for and expectation of confidentiality is entirely reasonable. All the more reason to understand what the therapist intends to do *before* he or she comes on board.

We've read many articles and books that assert fairly low recovery rates: somewhere in the range of 30%-40% may fully recover (depending on the definition used for recovery); another 40% or so remain in a marginal arena where they sustain only a minimal level of health but are consumed by their obsessive thoughts and are often miserable from the isolation their behaviors promote; another 5%-10% (or more) die from the effects of anorexia. We can't verify these percentages, and we always encourage others to do their own study in this area, but it is important to ask therapists what they believe are the likely results of treatment, and which modalities offer, in their view, the highest chance for success. There is research data currently available pointing to a much higher chance for recovery for adolescents—i.e., the Maudsley method. We recommend becoming familiar with this and asking the therapist you choose about Maudsley; if he or she doesn't use it, what is the reasoning behind that?

One thing is indisputable: Anorexia is incredibly difficult to treat. No one treatment model works with all patients, and it's unclear even which psychotherapy models work best with each age group. It's safe to say, though, that if the beliefs about the etiology of your child's illness are inaccurate or based on "old school" assumptions, and the treatment methods are based on inaccuracies, the treatment may not only be unhelpful, it could be downright harmful if lack of progress allows the anorexia more time to become further entrenched. You may not "know" the cause of your child's anorexia, but your intimate knowledge of your child and your gut instincts should not be dismissed. You are the "expert" on your particular child. If the therapist's views don't jibe with your instincts, if they aren't familiar with the latest research findings, finding someone else may save you and your child considerable agony—and may, in the long run, be the difference in saving your child, period.

Common Therapeutic Approaches

Other than the Maudsley method (which is described below), the common thread with these approaches seems to be the concept of the feedback loop— that is: If clients can access, with the help of a trained clinician, the emotional underpinnings of their illnesses, and learn how their unhealthy choices (restricting food) are holding them back from living healthy lives, then they will realize they have to make different choices (they have to eat), and then will be able to climb the ladder to health, unshackled by their burdens.

The key question here is whether this approach is sufficient with this illness, especially knowing that psychological factors are only one of a few factors in this illness. Before you tackle that question, you'll want to be familiar with some of the common approaches used by therapists and psychologists in treating anorexia:

- Psychodynamic
- Interpersonal
- Cognitive-behavioral
- Humanistic
- Family therapy
- Family-Based Treatment (also known as the Maudsley method, not to be confused with family therapy), OR . . .
- some combination of the above.

The psychodynamic approach assumes that the person struggling with anorexia is engaged in an individual struggle of powerlessness, and is trying to recapture some form of control over her life. Problems are assumed to be intra-psychic and unconscious, often stemming from and/or arising in childhood. The goal of this therapy is to increase self-awareness and understanding of how past issues and situations influence present-day behavior. This technique is open-ended, and to our knowledge has not been studied for effectiveness in those with anorexia in terms of sustaining recovery.

Interpersonal therapy (IPT) is another approach commonly used. It is based in the belief that problems occur in the context of relationships, and that these relationships have to be fixed in order for the problems to go away. What is interesting to note here is that it is almost universal that relationships are affected and become immensely dysfunctional around anorexic behaviors; what is not clear is whether dysfunctional relationships are part of the etiology of the illness for a given patient. Especially tricky is establishing a baseline of truth with the therapist. It is well known that eating disorders cause cognitive distortions, and that the egosyntonic nature of the illness (i.e., the merging of the anorexic beliefs and behaviors with the sufferer's identity and consequent desire to protect it from being taken away) causes sufferers to lie. Given that, how is a therapist to understand where reality lies if they don't seek or welcome information from the entire family? If all the therapist has to go on is what the client says, much of the work toward recovery will be a waste of precious time. If the therapist you choose assumes dysfunctional relationships are part of the root cause of the illness, it is crucial to ensure that they welcome and will seek out information from the family, at the beginning of treatment. We didn't know to ask this up front—in fact, we assumed they would want to know, as it only makes sense to us—but most didn't seek it out and were highly resistant when we offered input. They relied solely on what our daughter—who was clearly in the grips of her distorted ED mind—said.

Cognitive Behavior Therapy (CBT) has received the most attention from researchers. It is an approach that assumes cognitions (i.e., knowledge gained from perception, intuition and reasoning) are responsible for feelings and maladaptive behavior, and if those cognitions can be shifted, improved behavior will follow. This approach is known to be helpful in providing tools for those with eating disorders generally, but the egosyntonic nature of anorexia in particular—and thus the difficulty in generating alternate cognitions—severely limits CBT's effectiveness. Contrary to psychodynamic or interpersonal therapy, both of which are open-ended in duration, CBT aims to be time-limited—the average number of sessions being about 16 (but can vary according to the severity of the patient), and uses a didactic approach, i.e., a structured formula and homework assignments. Some therapists who offer outpatient therapy use CBT; others use some form of CBT combined with other approaches. We have never fully understood what that means, especially if CBT is a well-defined course. It is often part of the treatment program offered in residential, partial hospitalization (PHP) day programs or intensive outpatient (IOP) programs.

The humanistic approach to therapy is rooted in the belief that patients need to actualize their true potential in search of a meaningful existence. Within this approach, there is Dialectical Behavior Therapy (DBT), which combines CBT with mindfulness training, and Acceptance and Commitment Therapy (ACT), which believes that fighting against problems only perpetuates them or makes them worse; instead, according to this approach, finding ways to *accept* "what is" enables one to live more fully.

More recent therapies are proving helpful in dealing with anorexia. One is Cognitive Remediation Therapy [CRT], which is a time-specific program designed to address the cognitive inflexibilities in set shifting, etc., common to those with anorexia. Very few therapists with whom we spoke had even heard of CRT. As of this writing, a manual is being developed by Dr. Kathleen Kara Fitzpatrick at Stanford University. If this is an approach of interest to the reader, we recommend contacting Dr. Kathleen Fitzpatrick for the latest information on how to find a therapist who offers CRT.
Yet another therapy that is being developed, and which we have heard can be effective after a patient has been discharged from residential treatment, is Exposure and Response Prevention Therapy [ERPT]. This approach is designed to address the fears that may persist even after a successful stay in residential care, and may be helpful in reducing the all-too-common potential for relapse. For more information on ERPT, contact Professor Joanna Steinglass, MD, at Columbia University. Following is a link for a related article published by Gurze Press:
http://www.eatingdisordersreview.com/print/nl_edr_22_5print.html.

Other than in CRT or ERPT, which aim either to expand cognitive elasticity or deal with pathological fear, there is a commonly held belief in many of the modalities employed: If a therapist can help a client identify what is worth living for, help connect the client with her true inner self, and guide her toward working through difficulties in communication, this will reinforce the client's desire to live, which will help regain the strength to overcome the urge to restrict food intake. Surely, increasing self-awareness is an important part of the recovery process, but it alone cannot solve malnutrition.

All psychotherapeutic models are limited if the underlying belief of the treatment professionals is that the illness is primarily an emotionally driven illness. While any of the treatment modalities may be helpful in developing insight, and may assist in developing a sense of self (which in an anorexic has been decreased either before or as a result of the malnutrition), psychotherapy alone doesn't directly address the biological aspect of the illness, i.e., the effect anorexia has on the structure and function of the brain, which can only be corrected with *sustained nutrition.* Starvation itself causes irrational thought, psychosis, and depression. It causes or exacerbates obsessive-compulsive behaviors and generalized anxiety. Reversing this process requires nutritional restoration first and foremost. If your child is to receive treatment in a traditional outpatient setting (i.e., not using the Maudsley approach described below, and not be in residential or programs with meal supervision), the nutritional restoration component will usually be addressed by a nutritionist—the third member of the collaborative team, alongside the physician and therapist. As an outpatient, the client may see a nutritionist once per week, on average. Anorexia patients often report food consumption to the nutritionist, but at stages of the illness that are characterized by a lack of commitment to recovery, they are prone to exaggerate what they have consumed. It helps to understand that such "lying" is *a means of self-preservation* to someone in the grips of this disorder, and it is quite common. If possible, ask the nutritionist how this issue will be addressed; the answer may help you determine if the nutritionist will be strong enough to combat the eating disorder. If not, you may want to choose someone else, or perhaps consider a higher level of care, where meals are supervised. It may help you determine whether the Maudsley method, in which all meals are supervised (by you!) might be a better way to attack this problem.

At the time our daughter's treatment team consisted of a nutritionist, doctor and therapist, the therapist's report that she was making "significant improvement" only served to dismay us, because those reports didn't jibe with that we saw and experienced: precipitous weight loss, depression, edginess and hostility. She couldn't afford to lose more weight, and in spite of her "progress" in psychotherapy, she was still having trouble feeding herself adequately. Her body dysmorphia was in high gear; in short: "Progress" in the therapist's office wasn't translating into her being able to put food in her mouth. Thus, we found the feedback loop faulty—it couldn't become a closed loop UNTIL she became somewhat weight restored. This meant leaving school (again) for five months to enter residential treatment, followed by full day treatment (otherwise known as PHP—Partial Hospitalization Program), and then a half-day program (otherwise referred to as IOP—Intensive Outpatient Program). As she became weight restored in residential treatment, the anorexic indignation began to lose hold, and therapy began to gain some traction.

The Maudsley Method

The Maudsley program, also known as FBT (or Family-Based Treatment—not to be confused with family therapy, described above) is another approach to treating eating disorders that we did not know about until it was too late. In FBT, parents are enlisted as a crucial component of the team, and refeeding is the primary goal at the beginning. We will provide a more detailed overview of the Maudsley method below, and we would encourage everyone to become familiar with it, as it is an *evidence-based approach* that is yielding far higher recovery rates than traditional methods. Being an evidence-based approach means that there have been randomized controlled trials comparing the Maudsley method with other forms of treatment. Research results show that two-thirds of patients are recovered at the end of FBT, and 75%-80% are weight restored at a five-year follow up, with marked improvement in psychological factors as well.

This, of course, is far more encouraging than the 30%-40% recovery results we hear from the more common approaches above. Unfortunately, however, the Maudsley approach is aimed specifically at *adolescents living at home*, and therefore isn't usually appropriate for college-aged students or young adults (or older) not living at home. It also may not be effective for those who have been struggling with this illness for too long before treatment began. What is the Maudsley method? And how does it fit into the timeline of theories regarding etiology and treatment of this disorder? Let's first consider a very short (and necessarily incomplete) history of the field of anorexia pre-Maudsley:

In the 1870s, when anorexia nervosa was first named, physicians theorized that families were to blame and should therefore be removed from the patient's surroundings in order to effectively treat the patient. In 1947, Dr. John Berkman at the Mayo Clinic attributed starvation to disturbances in clients' relationships with parents. Psychological theories variously describe anorexia as a defense against emerging sexuality, difficulty separating from parents, and enmeshed family dynamics. In the 1960s, Salvador Minuchin and Mara Selvine Palazzoli theorized that abnormal family dynamics—characterized by rigidity, enmeshment, conflict avoidance, and parental over-involvement—were a major factor in the development of the disorder, but also concluded these were not necessarily *causes* of the illness. They developed family therapy (not to be confused with Family-Based Therapy; i.e., Maudsley) as a treatment methodology to address abnormal family interactions.

In the early 1970s, a leading therapist named Hilde Bruch, in her book *The Golden Cage*, postulated that the pursuit of thinness developed in a social context in which the role, status and image of women was in flux. Her view was that the drive for thinness was the anorexic's failed attempt at autonomy. She saw it as a desperate fight against feeling enslaved and exploited, and represented a misguided path to independence. Other theories have included the beliefs that anorexia results from a fear of becoming orally impregnated or a response to deep-seated distrust—this latter belief postulated by none other than Dr. Steven Levenkrom, the psychologist who treated Karen Carpenter.

All such theories have a weak empirical foundation, as very few studies have been conducted to prove or disprove them. They are merely ideas formulated in an attempt to make sense of this confounding illness. Furthermore, these hypotheses were developed before the advent of the technologies (PET scans and MRIs) that have allowed researchers to see inside the brain—a development spearheaded by UC San Diego's Dr. Walter Kaye, among others, and before the study of genetics showed a genetic underpinning that makes certain people vulnerable to developing eating disorders. Nonetheless, outdated theories continue to inform the choice of treatment approaches used by many providers today.

Since Minuchin's "psychosomatic theory" of the family was postulated, many studies have been conducted to see if there are common characteristics in families of anorexic patients, and—not surprisingly—what has been found is that families of anorexic patients are quite heterogeneous with regard to the nature of the relationships within the family, the emotional climate in the family, and patterns of interaction. (See 'Family Interventions in Adolescent Anorexia Nervosa,' by Daniel le Grange, PhD and Ivan Eisler, PhD. In Child Adolescent Psychiatric Clin N. Am 18 (2008) 159-173.)

As a result of this knowledge, there has been a shift in the context of the development of the eating disorder—from seeing the family as a cause to seeing the family as part of a dynamic gone awry (a dynamic which may or may not function to sustain the illness), to a more explicit non-blaming approach in which the family is now seen as a resource to help the adolescent in the process of recovery. In addition, with brain imaging and genetic studies in just the last 12 years or so, experts have a greater understanding of the differences in the brain structure and function of anorexics compared to the non-anorexic population.

Unfortunately, however, not all practitioners have kept up with the research or have incorporated the latest evidence-based results into their treatment choices. One often hears of parents who are marginalized and excluded from communicating with treatment teams. Patients who are resistant to or ambivalent about recovery can easily manipulate a treatment team into believing the family is the problem, which drives a wedge between those most invested in seeing their loved ones recover.

The Maudsley Approach (Family-Based Treatment or FBT)

In the late 1970s and early 1980s, Drs. Christopher Dare, Ivan Eisler, Gerald Russell, and George Szmulker, who worked with eating disordered patients at the Institute of Psychiatry at the Maudsley Hospital in London, developed a new form of family-based therapy aimed at supporting and empowering families in the effort to eliminate anorexia in their children.

In 1986, Dr. Daniel Le Grange, of the University of Chicago, joined the research team at Maudsley, and introduced it to his colleagues at Stanford University, including Dr. James Lock. LeGrange and Lock collaborated on studying the Maudsley approach. Their research showed that 90% of adolescents who received the Maudsley treatment recovered or made significant gains; five years later, 90 percent had fully recovered. In 2000, Drs. Lock and LeGrange published a treatment manual on the Maudsley approach.

The Maudsley approach works in three phases, taking place over the course of approximately one year, during which a therapist meets with the family approximately 15 to 20 times. An essential tenet of the Maudsley approach is that neither the parents nor the afflicted child are to blame for the onset of the illness. Searching for the causes of the illness is suspended until nutritional restoration has been attained.

Below is a summary; more detailed information can be obtained from www.maudsleyparents.org.

Maudsley Phase I: Weight restoration
During the first phase, the goal is weight restoration. Parents take charge of providing all meals and snacks for their child. The therapist's role during this phase is to remind the patient and family of the dangers of malnutrition associated with anorexia, which include, among other things, hypothermia, growth hormone changes, cardiac dysfunction, and cognitive and emotional changes. Parents express sympathy with their child's predicament but consistently and persistently insist that starvation is not an option. The message that is communicated is, essentially, if this were cancer, chemo would be required to save your life, even if the chemo makes you feel horrible in the

short-term. For this illness, food *is* the medicine. The effect of refeeding an anorexic may be as discomfiting as chemo is to a cancer patient, but both are necessary for recovery.

To one who has not experienced anorexia, that may sound like an implausible comparison: How can eating be as uncomfortable as enduring chemotherapy? Precisely because eating is the enemy of anorexia. For someone in the grips of anorexia, eating provokes extreme anxiety (emotionally and physiologically); it is scary, repulsive, and greatly discomforting to someone under the sway of the disorder. The seeming illogic of this is among the most difficult things for family and friends to comprehend and deal with.

We've heard horror stories of parents trying to manage this phase: the anorexic child refusing to ingest breakfast for an entire day while the parents remain at the table, calmly outwaiting the child; plates being dumped on the floor or thrown across the room; horrific and sustained tantrums; bolts being installed on doors and windows to prevent the child from running away. The degree of unification between parents required to make this phase work is obvious: If either one gives in, the effort will be lost. Parents not only have to be on the same page at all times, but they have to recite the same words, in unison. Not an easy task for most couples, even those with the best relationships.

We've heard of parents having to take leaves of absence from work to manage this scenario at the worst of times. The main point is, nothing the child wants—cell phone, computer, time with friends, school—nothing else is allowed to happen until meals are eaten. If breakfast doesn't get consumed until late night, lunch and dinner will still have to follow, no matter what the hour. It can be an agonizing few months.

Phase II: Returning control of eating to the adolescent
The second phase of Maudsley usually begins three to five months after the start of treatment, when the child has shown acceptance of the parental demand that food be consumed, when there has been steady weight gain, and when the mood of the family has shifted—i.e., when the eating disorder has been strong-armed into submission, to some degree. During this second phase, the patient is encouraged to take more control of preparing his or her meals. In addition, the emotional, psychological and communication issues relative to the parent-adolescent relationship can be initiated. This is postponed until there has been nutritional rehabilitation because the belief is that during the acute state of the illness—such as during the first phase of

treatment—the mind, rendered irrational by malnutrition, can't assimilate or make use of psychological insights. Placing the focus on psychotherapy or family therapy before nutritional restoration has occurred, according to adherents of this treatment model, *only serves to reinforce the adversarial relationship on which the eating disorder thrives.* This belief is key to this therapy, an important point we will address later.

Phase III: Establishing healthy adolescent identity
The third phase is initiated when self-starvation has abated and the adolescent is able to maintain 95% of ideal weight. The focus of treatment starts to shift to the impact anorexia has had on the individual's effort to establish a healthy adolescent identity. This entails a review of central issues of adolescence, including increased personal autonomy for the adolescent, the development of appropriate parental boundaries, and the need for the parents to reorganize their life together after their children's expected departure to college or an independent adult life.

For more details on the Maudsley approach, please refer to books by Dr. James Lock on the topic. The websites www.maudsleyparents.org and www.feast-ed.org are excellent sources of support and information, as are the eating disorder programs at the University of Chicago, Stanford University and University of California San Diego.

Our story, continued:

We quickly understood that the Maudsley method would not work with our daughter. For one thing, she was already an adult, living away from home, desperate to establish her independence from us. Some people felt that her refusal to live at home during this time was entirely her eating disorder talking—being at home for her was tantamount to submitting to treatment and recovery on our terms. We felt, however, that her repugnance at the thought of being at home had components of both her eating disorder and her healthy self struggling for autonomy. Feeling coerced could have dire results. We wanted to squelch her eating disorder, but the roots of the eating disorder and the roots of her healthy attempt at individuation were so entangled that we feared pulling out the weed would destroy the plant. Clearly, the developmental stage of young adulthood, along with the practical aspects of being away at college or living an independent adult life, makes addressing the eating disorder via the Maudsley approach extremely difficult. Secondly, our daughter's social problems in our home town would have made it impossible for us to get her here, as she was disconnected from her old friends—indeed, friendships that had been extremely challenging for her throughout high school. Being back here, confronted by what she perceived as her social failures, was simply too difficult emotionally. She would have no one she felt good about to spend time with, and she certainly didn't want to be around us, since we were at war with her eating disorder, which she felt she needed; in fact, she *was* her anorexia, then. She was not someone who could externalize her disorder; it was already engrained in who she was trying to become.

Thirdly, and most importantly, she was defiantly convinced that we were at the root of her problems. We believed otherwise, as we had been endlessly reflecting on every aspect of our role as parents, reviewing every interaction that had any relevance along the course of her life. But having been hijacked by this eating disorder, she was incapable of perceiving that we weren't what was controlling her. And, if the Maudsley method involved our controlling her food intake, then there would be no way we could EVER convince her that we weren't—and never had been—controlling her.

We were devastated beyond words at our helplessness to employ the treatment modality that demonstrated the greatest potential for recovery. But even if we couldn't be the agent of change in terms of refeeding her, we certainly hoped that her treatment team could find a way to restore her weight as the first priority of treatment. If the research was showing that nutritional and weight restoration causes changes in the brain chemistry that reduces depression, irrational thoughts, and cognitive distortions, then even if we couldn't be the ones to refeed her, surely the treatment team could help devise a plan based on the same premise as the Maudsley approach: focus on nutritional restoration first, and *then* address emotional issues.

Unfortunately, nothing could have been further from the truth. Our daughter's first outpatient treatment team, as well as many of her other teams in residential, PHP, and IOP care, seemed to believe that anorexia is primarily an emotional disorder, not a disorder of the brain, and therefore directed treatment at uncovering the psychological problems and working out issues in talk therapy, rather than focusing on refeeding as a way to recalibrate the dysregulations in the neurotransmitters in her brain that were in part causing her to restrict. Some were simply unaware of the recent research studies indicating the efficacy of the Maudsley approach, or understood what the Minnesota Starvation Study indicated were the simple behavioral and psychological effects of malnutrition. The treatment teams we thought we had carefully chosen (back when we'd had to make decisions before we knew what we were up against) didn't ascribe to the current knowledge that anorexic behaviors are caused in part by complex biological processes, and that the resulting starvation and malnutrition further exacerbates disordered thoughts and behaviors. That the most essential factor in treating her anorexia would be food, and lots of it, seemed not to be part of the initial equation by the specialists attending to our daughter.

Three months after we first found a treatment team, during which time her weight plummeted to dangerously low levels, we were initially relieved to have finally gotten her into a residential treatment facility. By that time, in spite of her team's reassurance that they knew what they were doing, and their admonition for us to back off and let them do their jobs, our daughter was delusional and irrational, and her heart rate so low that a second physician who examined her wanted to hospitalize her immediately. The only reason the doctor didn't insist on hospitalization at that point was the fear of losing the single opening at a residential facility that we'd heard was coming up shortly. Residential care aims to accomplish refeeding while addressing the psychological and other aspects of the disorder—whereas hospitalization is designed only to stabilize physical symptoms. Also, insurance often covers hospitalization only until a patient reaches 75% of her healthy weight; patients are often discharged when they are still extremely ill. Thus, risking a few days outside the hospital setting in order to be available to claim the bed in the residential treatment center, offered the best long-term solution. Those few interim days were agonizing, to put it mildly. We were afraid of her heart giving out, of her dying in her sleep. She wanted to drive the car—yet another indication of her inability to grasp how grave her situation had become; many arguments and recriminations ensued. We felt how much she despised us, when all we were trying to do was keep her alive until help could be arranged.

The residential facility we were waiting on was chosen based on somewhat limited information, given the short time frame we had since discovering our daughter's problem; we thought at the time that we had done substantial research, but we didn't know what we didn't know. The founder of that facility is a well-known and outspoken therapist, who discloses to her clients and the world that she herself has fully recovered from anorexia. We thought this would be inspirational to our daughter. In addition, we read three books she authored, and her books made sense to us at the time. We felt that our research efforts had paid off, and we were glad not to be in a position to have to blindly follow someone else's advice with regard to which residential facility to utilize.

It turns out we didn't have nearly enough information at the time, and of course we had not yet arrived at an understanding of the chasm between research and practice. The eating disorder guru at the helm of that first facility handled our daughter (and us) in what now seems the worst possible way.

An adult (a person 18 years or older) entering residential treatment has the freedom to walk out; these are not locked facilities (the same is true of hospitals with eating disorder units). Unless adult patients are admitted to psychiatric units on a "72–hour hold" (what is commonly called a "5150" for the penal code that authorizes the state to hold people against their will if they are a danger to themselves or others), they are free to leave at any time. And knowing our daughter as we do, we were sure she would leave the moment things got uncomfortable for her, if she could. Why would she stay when this residential option was clearly not her choice? When she hadn't even yet admitted she *had* a problem? When, even after acknowledging it, she demonstrated she wasn't willing to give it up? She was going to be "a tough nut to crack," everyone knew, because from the moment one enters residential treatment, eating-disordered behaviors are not tolerated. Patients must eat, period. Some places offer supplements if the food isn't eaten; others send them to hospitals for inpatient treatment. But they must eat. So we knew this was going to be rough. She couldn't do it on her own; the voice in her head (or whatever each individual calls it) wouldn't let her. She needed this level of help, but was bitterly unhappy that we had forced her to get it. We used the only leverage we had to get her into residential care and to comply with her treatment team: We told her that our continuing to pay for her college education was conditional on her getting well; that she must follow the recommendations of her physicians, who were saying residential care was indicated, and that she must stay until the treatment team in the residential facility determined that she was well enough to leave. In essence, we made it clear she must complete the program. To her, this felt like blackmail. It would be hard to argue otherwise, but to us, it was our only way to ensure compliance, as we knew how important academics were (and are) to her. Though we ached for the pain she was suffering, we were relieved that she was at last going to get fed, in a safe environment.

Four days after entering residential, she called home defiantly asserting that she just realized she's 18 and that no one can make her stay. She blamed us for deceiving her by not telling her that she didn't *have* to agree to being admitted; in fact, she'd been telling everyone at the facility that she'd been forced into the decision. She even claimed she no longer gave a damn about her education; she had had enough, it was intolerable, and she was going to leave.

We frantically contacted everyone on her treatment team, as well as professionals in our local area and on her previous outpatient treatment team. We told the residential staff not to give her the cash we had to supply upon admission (for use on outings), that she had no place to go to (as she had already given up her dorm room at school and we wouldn't allow her to come home and starve herself to death). She had no money, no car, and no place to live. In addition, she learned that if she were to bolt without providing a two-week notice, the facility would not refund the $4,000 deposit we'd had to submit—money that had been earmarked for her sister's college education. Somehow, the crisis passed and she didn't bolt.

Nevertheless, she soon began in earnest devising a plan to leave with a two-week notice. We reiterated to the staff that our daughter had no safe place to go. They assured us they wouldn't let her leave unless she had a safe plan. Without one, we were told, she would likely be picked up by local police and escorted to the nearest psych unit on a 72-hour hold. At that point, we were even starting to investigate conservatorship, as clearly she was not able to make rational decisions about her medical care. We kept reminding the director of the facility that they held the key to keeping her there, as our daughter knew that she would not be able to leave until such time as the treatment team felt she was well enough to be released.

But then, against our wishes, the director of the facility abruptly informed us that she and our daughter had made an agreement: Once she reached her first weight goal, and could maintain it for two weeks, she could leave the facility and return to college!

We were stunned. We knew her first weight goal was still so low as to qualify as anorexic in the DSM IV; on weight alone, she still met the criteria for hospitalization! We had by this time come to understand that the brain can't recalibrate until sometime after the body reaches *normal* weight. We pleaded with them to tell her that she wasn't ready to function outside of residential until she could at least reach a second weight goal. This, we hoped, would give her brain time to absorb the nutrition, and possibly soften her defiant hold on the anorexia, or the deathly grip it had on her. And, even if her defiance persisted at a higher weight, it would buy critical time. Many people in residential treatment gain the minimum weight required for discharge, but then resolve to lose all they've gained the minute they get out. We knew there was a good chance our daughter would do the same thing. But there was also a chance she wouldn't. Even if she did, she would at least have some padding, a buffer to buy us time. If they let her go at the first weight goal, there would be no buffer.

If they let her out being severely underweight, she'd have virtually no chance to overcome the anorexia on her own with only outpatient care. In her college town, there are no day programs or even half-day programs. How could returning to the same level of care she had left in order to enter residential treatment, when she lost over 20% of her body weight in just a few short months prior to entering residential, bring about any positive outcome?

In addition, we were fortunate that our secondary insurance carrier seemed willing to go the distance with regard to treatment—a rarity in this field, where so many patients are forcibly discharged by insurance companies saying they won't foot the bill any longer, in spite of treatment professionals insisting that the patients are not strong enough to avoid immediate relapse upon discharge.

But the facility director insisted that our daughter was intransigent (no surprise to us); our daughter refused to cooperate in her therapy; she was resistant to the treatment strategy; she didn't trust anyone, etc. We asked them to hold off on any expectation that she willingly participate in therapy sessions until more time had passed. (Maudsley research has shown that the brain can't take in all the therapy until body weight is restored and the brain has a chance to recalibrate.) We begged them to keep her until she recovered enough to be *able* to participate. But the director asserted that the only way to get our daughter to begin trusting anyone with whom she might seek treatment in the future would be to abide by her desire to leave. She said there was a good chance she would fail once discharged (duh!) and if she did, she would return to them "with her tail between her legs" and be more compliant.

Their rationale stunned us, once again. They were treating her anorexia as if it was purely an emotional issue, to be solved primarily with psychotherapy, and not a biological illness that has to be corrected first and foremost with sustained refeeding! Plus, they didn't know our daughter; otherwise they'd have known this is someone who has never, ever done anything with her tail between her legs. Her stubbornness and her refusal to admit she was wrong about something were the stuff of legend in our family. We cajoled; we pleaded; but she wouldn't listen. She was the expert and we were merely parents who were clueless as to how the process worked. *Let the professionals do their job!* (This was a dismissive mantra we would hear often from our daughter over the ensuing months, but more about that later.)

After we lost this first skirmish—of whether to keep her in residential or let her leave—we focused on the next battle. If the treatment team refused to say that they felt she wasn't ready to go and our daughter persisted in obtaining her discharge at such a low weight, then we would at least make sure she enter a PHP full-day program, so that she could continue to have the majority of her meals monitored, and get the nutritional and additional guidance we felt she needed during the transition from residential to private life: help with eating, cooking, grocery shopping, and later perhaps dealing with her complicated feelings about food, etc.

Incredibly, the facility director again disagreed. She felt she needed to comply with our daughter's strong wish to return to her college life, where only minimal supervision—a weekly appointment with a physician and therapist, and a couple group meetings with the nutritionist—was available.

When we realized we were losing this battle as well, we immediately contacted the nutritionist to request as many supervised meals as they could offer. All they could arrange was one or two supported meals each week. This is a huge change from the 42 meals/snacks provided in a residential setting.

In addition, she would be returning to school in the summer, when friendships would be even harder for a person plagued by social anxiety to find than during the school year. In short: They were relegating her to a deadly combination: isolation, and inadequate support. Exactly the kind of environment an eating disorder thrives on!

We were immensely disappointed with the therapist who chose to collude with our daughter's eating disorder rather than support us in overpowering her disorder. (Incidentally, at a later point in her recovery, our daughter admitted that her eating disorder had been able to survive for so long because everybody, including us, *kept giving her an out.* This is a critical insight: Perhaps she was actually hoping desperately to find someone strong enough to overpower the eating disorder by simply taking charge, no matter how much she protested to the contrary.)

In spite of our deep concerns regarding our daughter's discharge from residential, and the staff's not insisting that she step down to a full-day or even a half-day program, the director said she intended to have our daughter write up a "binding contract" that she, the treatment team and we would have to sign before she could leave. We found out later that our daughter mistakenly believed we had initiated the creation of that contract, which fueled her anger toward us for quite some time. In any case, the bottom line of the contract was that if she lost more than two pounds and didn't regain it within one week, she would have to reenter residential treatment, without argument.

They were consigning her to Hell. We knew it, and were powerless to prevent it because we couldn't make her stay in treatment when her team was allowing her to leave! The contract seemed a sham, but it was all we had. Going along with it and establishing a new team for her to work with when she was back in school seemed our only option, and our only hope of saving her. This turned out to be a black-hole summer for her, and became an even worse autumn for us, followed by another "forced" stay in residential before we could begin to see even a glimmer of light at the end of that very long, very dark tunnel.

So, what are the takeaways from this chapter?

To summarize:

- Understanding that research study results aren't disseminated throughout the treatment community in a timely fashion, and that you may need to ascertain what the treatment team knows and believes before you enlist their help.

- In selecting a physician, ask about their expertise and experience in handling anorexia. What are their qualifications? What do they know, specifically, about the medical dangers, and what tests, at what frequency, will they administer? At what weight will the physician recommend a change to a higher level of care?

- If your pediatrician is not an expert, do not accept the assessment that "there's nothing wrong with your child." Ask for a referral to an eating disorder specialist.

- Alternately, skip the step of going to a general family pediatrician and start with a specialist in eating disorders. You can find them on many websites, some of which are listed in the resource chapter at the back of this book.

- Ask everyone on the team what their beliefs are regarding the etiology and best treatment methods, including *why* they believe what they do? Is refeeding an essential priority, at least in the beginning of treatment? How will weight stabilization and weight gain be addressed? If the illness progresses in spite of this level of treatment, what criteria will they use to recommend a higher level of care?

- Have a conversation with the therapist about what psychological interventions they employ, and whether you can expect to participate in family therapy.

- If your child requires residential treatment: Before you decide on a facility or recommend one to your child or to the treatment team, have a conversation with the staff of the facility about how they will respond if their clients choose to leave against medical advice (AMA); ask if they will abide by any expectations you may have of their treatment (such as we had: that she stay until she is weight-restored, even if she doesn't "participate" or "embrace" the individual and group therapy sessions she will be required to attend).

- If you agree patients have a better chance at recovery if they can gradually take the skills and knowledge learned in residential treatment and apply them in a step-down facility, rather than returning to their former life cold turkey, ask the staff at the facility what their policy is with regard to discharging to a step-down facility. In other words, if a patient resists going to PHP or IOP, will they allow her to skip this crucial step in treatment, during which support is gradually reduced *only as they demonstrate the ability to feed themselves*?

CHAPTER FIVE: FINDING AN OUTPATIENT TREATMENT TEAM THAT COMMUNICATES AND UNDERSTANDS LOOPHOLES

Something else we wish we had known at the beginning of this troubling journey was how critical it would be to make sure that the physician, nutritionist and therapist—who would come to make up our daughter's treatment team—would actually *work together as a team*, and that they clearly understood the function of loopholes in dealing with eating disordered clients.

In the beginning, when we were scrambling to address our daughter's problem, we had little time (and limited options) for choosing a treatment team: After contacting the only therapist in her college town with eating-disorder experience who responded to our initial, desperate email, we next made an appointment with the medical director at the university's student health center. The center assigned us a registered dietitian on staff—who quickly assessed that this case was out of her league, so we were directed to find a nutritionist at a local Intensive Outpatient Program (IOP). We already had learned there was only one IOP in the area, so we had little choice but to enlist that nutritionist (who co-owned the IOP) as the third member of our daughter's team.

We had no reason to imagine this trio of care providers wouldn't function *as a team*. At the very least, we were told they would communicate with one another regularly to maintain a coordinated plan with agreed-upon goals and contingencies, that they would "compare notes" on what took place during her appointments, and, if she wasn't showing improvement, they would let us know. What we found out, in the course of trying to understand their treatment rationale, was that they didn't communicate as often as we thought our daughter's case warranted, they didn't always agree on treatment strategies, and it was rarely ever clear who was taking the lead.

What we came to understand only much later was that most care providers in individual practice who accept insurance do not get reimbursed for the inordinate amount of time it takes outside of actual office visits to coordinate the patient's care. Due to their contracts with insurance companies, they can only charge fees in accordance with what insurance companies deem reasonable, and these only cover billable office visits.

As it turns out, many of the experts in the E.D. field choose not to work with insurance because it allows them the freedom to make decisions regarding care without having to be limited by what third party insurance representatives decide; it frees them up from endless hours of paperwork justifying the care they are providing; and it allows them to set prices they think are reasonable so that they can be reimbursed for the extensive time outside of office visits required to coordinate care with a team, in addition to office visits. This makes sense for all the reasons they choose to do this, both for themselves as well as for their patients, but lacking insurance coverage to cover these bills, many people are excluded from getting expert care. There are many stories of parents mortgaging or losing their homes, their entire retirement, and going into debt they have no ability to repay in order to provide care. Others have been unable to access care only to have their children die. This is a very serious problem.

On the other hand, IOPs are able to charge higher fees, as it established with insurance carriers that IOPs offer programs at a certain number of hours per week (e.g., 3-hour segments three times per week, etc.). IOPs, therefore, have flexibility to ensure they are compensated for their time spent communicating with family members and coordinating with the other members on the team, whether they are employees of their IOP or professionals in private practice in the communities and communicating with families.

What we found out when the bills came in was that our daughter's therapist and physician did not get paid for any time spent outside of our daughter's weekly office visit, and that the nutritionist at the IOP was compensated at a rate 10 times higher than the physician and therapist. She should have taken the lead, therefore, in fielding questions from us, incorporating information on our daughter's mental state (that we're sure she wouldn't allow to be shown when at her appointments) into a coordinated treatment plan, and communicating with us on a regular basis. This did not happen (and we would be surprised if the physician and therapist knew the discrepancy in their reimbursements).

This is not to say that the team didn't spend time responding to our inquiries or discussing among themselves how to treat our daughter. We know they did, but it was made clear on many occasions that they were going "above and beyond" in our daughter's case, and weren't exactly happy about it.

But as we communicated with our daughter by phone or in person and found out at times that she was spiraling out of control—information only we would know, knowing that she would hide that during her appointments with them—we often found they didn't want our input; they didn't want to deal with us. They often brushed our concerns aside, saying that we should trust them, that they were not going to let her fall through the cracks, and that they didn't have time to deal with us. They, after all, were the professionals. They were clearly annoyed with and felt put upon by us, and used that to craft a theory that our involvement in her care was indicative of how we must have been as parents prior to her illness, and seemed to decide that this may have caused her illness or at least and may have been a factor in maintaining her illness. Meanwhile, we were left in a constant state of bewilderment that those charged with her care weren't taking action. We just wanted some answers, like: Why were they allowing her to play collegiate sports, as she continued to lose weight and display increasingly bizarre and angry behavior, when we had read that she could die from a heart attack on the court. What was the rationale for having her on Prozac, when the studies we'd read about suggested *this was not helpful for anorexic patients in the acute stages of the illness*? Why not try other medications we'd read about that showed more promise? Why was she not being taken off birth control pills so they could determine with objective measures if she was amenhorreic? Wouldn't such objective data help persuade her to see the danger her body was in, which the other mechanisms of the illness were preventing her from seeing? Why were they allowing her to sink so low before they insisted on a higher level of treatment, when studies show the sooner anorexia is attacked aggressively, the better the chances for survival?

Clear communication with the treatment team, in our case (because she was 18, and therefore an adult under the law) was initially blocked by HIPAA laws—which are designed to protect patients' privacy but can result in shutting out those who are powerful advocates and a valuable resource (and who, by the way, are generally *paying for* the care). But even when that got sorted out (our daughter agreed, albeit not because she wanted to, to sign releases so the team could freely communicate with us), we were never told who was the leader of the team, which of them would regularly update us on behalf of the team, and if disagreements among them about the treatment plan came up, whose opinion would prevail.

The lack of an organized, coherent treatment strategy (and a clear plan to communicate about it) proved hugely problematic, especially when it seemed obvious to us that changing circumstances called for a recalibration of the plan. The first occurrence came near the end of second quarter in her freshman year; anticipating that she would be home for several weeks following finals, we felt strongly that she should see an ED-specialist physician while home so there wouldn't be a lapse in monitoring her physical condition (precarious as it still was). We searched for, and found, an ED specialist in our area, and suggested that her physician provide a referral for this interim care.

What happened next revealed an enormous and potentially deadly trap that we had not seen mentioned in any ED literature. Nonetheless it presented a major stumbling block in our efforts to get our daughter the care she needed. We have come to call it . . .

The ED Loophole

At this time, it was becoming clear to the physician that our daughter was failing miserably in the outpatient setting; her weight was plummeting, and the doctor was clearly disappointed in what the scales were saying. While at first she wasn't sure it was necessary to have our daughter see an ED-specialist at home to get weighed and have vital signs checked, the night before our daughter's return, we received a call from her advise us not only to set up that appointment here with the doctor we found, but also to admit our daughter to a residential care facility as soon as possible. She felt the second opinion would affirm and underscore her recommendation of residential care. It should be noted here that we were left to our own devices to find an appropriate residential care center. Not having a list of residential facilities to refer to is probably an indication of the level of a primary caregiver's ED expertise, and in retrospect we wish we had known that. We would recommend that you ask any provider you are considering entrusting your child's life with where they refer their clients if their situations require more intensive care, and then take that list and investigate on your own, or perhaps if they can't tell you places they recommend and why, to consider finding other, perhaps more qualified, care givers.

When we got this call from the doctor, we spoke with the nutritionist on the team (co-owner of the IOP) and her opinion conflicted with the doctor's recommendation. She felt residential wasn't necessary just yet – though probably would be soon – and that she could string our daughter along maybe another week or two to try to gain her trust sufficient to get her to eat; she suggested increasing IOP care to 5 days per week so she could stay in school (even though her facility didn't offer 5 days per week care!). Given the drastic weight loss over the previous 12 weeks, we had no indication (and even less confidence) that the nutritionist would gain any traction with her. This dichotomy in the recommendations of key members of the treatment team was astonishing to us. It basically created a massive loophole that *our daughter would have defiantly waltzed right through*, had we not aggressively plugged it in the few hours we had before she arrived home.

Loopholes are what eating disorders thrive on. They are chinks in the armor, holes in the safety net. People with eating disorders are keenly able to detect them; eating disordered thoughts require them to stay alive and continue wreaking havoc. In our daughter's case, since residential treatment was akin to prison, and the forced change from a known environment to something completely unknown was frightening; given a choice, she would have done just about anything to avoid the unknown and stay where she was.

In short: It is absolutely essential that every member of the treatment team not only be reading out of the same book, but reading the same words from the same page, in unison. If the treatment team isn't in agreement, the treatment members should agree and it should be made clear from the outset whose professional advice will prevail when decisions need to be made, with the acknowledgement that all providers need to get behind it. Anything less creates potential loopholes that undermine even the best treatment efforts.

Our daughter's doctor wanted her to be in residential care. Clearly she was failing in outpatient care, given her continued weight loss and the increase in erratic behavior. Medically she had a number of problems that were nearing danger levels. How is it that the nutritionist could think things would be okay? And how could she justify asserting her opinion, which contradicted the doctor's? How could she not see the loophole created by doing so? Providers who don't understand the danger of loopholes are not, in our opinion, qualified to treat eating-disordered clients. It should be the very <u>first</u> lesson taught in "Eating Disorders 101."

Differences of opinions among the team members created one of the many Catch-22's we would encounter in our two-year odyssey: We had made it clear to our daughter that she had to follow her team's advice, so what were we to do when the team wasn't acting in unison?

Frantically, we drafted a letter to the team insisting that someone had to be the leader. Aside from the enormous problem of our daughter having the opportunity to choose not to go to residential, the lack of consensus put us in a position of having to choose which professional to side with. Choosing one over the other could have been disastrous in the future by creating dysfunctional alliances, among other things. In the nick of time, the nutritionist capitulated and agreed with the doctor's recommendations. The message our daughter finally heard was that her entire team felt she must step up to the highest level of care, and this was reinforced by the ED specialist physician she had to see while at home on her break from school.

This was not the only instance of inadequate teamwork. We experienced it at several critical junctures, involving different teams. After her first stint in residential, when she was let out prematurely (in spite of our desperate pleas to the contrary), she was allowed to return to her college town on a "contract" she developed at the advice of her therapist, which specified she would have to reenter residential if she lost more than a few pounds and didn't get back into her "safe weight zone" within a week or two. With a new physician, who we were told was "the best there was" in that town—and who had been recommended by the nutritionist and worked well with the therapist she continued to see—we had reason to believe the team would work together this time. The team members knew each other and worked together on other cases. Little did we know how dangerous the ED landscape would prove to be.

Out of residential, within a short time her weight had dropped below the agreed-upon threshold. When the doctor didn't take action, we were shocked and dismayed, to say the least. What use is a contract, especially when the limits get tested the first time, if it isn't going to be enforced, and when the doctor in outpatient – who isn't even connected with the residential team – doesn't even believe in contracts? We couldn't expect our daughter to take it seriously if the team didn't! Now it became just a game (but a game with deadly consequences): Because our daughter saw that no one would hold her to the agreement, she kept pushing the envelope (and getting away with it), which only served to reinforce her eating disordered thought process. Her team wasn't holding her accountable, so she felt she couldn't be all that bad! At various points we had been strongly cautioned to "back off and let the team manage the case," "allow her to take responsibility for her recovery," and "don't overreact at every indication that things may not be going right." Recovery is not on straight trajectory, we were reminded; it's a one-step-forward, two-steps-back kind of thing. So, we bit our lips and agreed to one brief weekly email from the physician with three data points: whether she had lost weight and was in the danger zone (no specific numbers would be provided), her pulse, and her blood pressure. After another week of her being below contract weight, we couldn't stand it any more. We phoned and asked: With all due respect, *what is going on?* At what point is our daughter going to be told she has to go back to residential, now that she is convinced she can ignore the contract? They kept giving her one more week, and one more week. She was playing them for the fools they seemed to be. Several weeks went by, and finally the team agreed she should be in residential. The new loophole became their not having held her to the contract when it counted most; our daughter thus had sufficient time to come up with arguments against going into residential that were hard to oppose. She agreed that she had fallen short of the contract goal, but argued persuasively that she'd made a dramatic turnaround in the past week, and that she had just started to make new friends with whom she was able to eat meals. She begged us not to take these gains away . . .

We wouldn't have been faced with this if the doctor had sent our daughter back to residential when she didn't live up to the contract in the first place. Now we were confronted with an impossible decision: If we ignored her plea and sent her back to residential, it would risk the newly developed friendships (which we had long desperately wanted for her, and which might have helped her overcome her depression and create the desire to fight this illness), it would be to dismiss the gains she had made just made, and perhaps worst of all, it would convey to her that we didn't believe she had turned the corner on her recovery. It felt like we would be punishing her! At the same time, we were concerned that *we were now the ones being played for the fool.* To some extent, we were being held hostage by our fear: If we overrode her pleas and sent her back, she would be so angry that she could easily dig her heels in and become even more entrenched in her illness, just to spite us. The eating disorder seemed firmly in control of all of us, and whatever we decided seemed fraught with danger.

We came up with a counter proposal: A choice to either go back into residential, which everyone except her felt would provide the best chance of being able to return to school in the fall, or agree to a new contract. However, this time we would create a contract that would include *weekly weight gain goals* intended to get her to a healthy level in time for fall quarter. We knew she'd choose the contract rather than go back to residential at this point, and we were also fairly certain she wouldn't be able to meet such substantial weekly goals. We felt that her likely inability to meet these goals would end up getting her back into residential treatment, which would get her the help she needed to be safe, and it offered her choice, which seemed critical for her at this stage of her development.

Everyone went along with this compromise, even her doctor (reluctantly). Nonetheless, this period proved to be among the most stressful we had yet endured. Our daughter was furious that we had "blackmailed" her into choosing a new contract that we wrote. Each week we were calling residential centers trying to gauge anticipated openings, convinced she wouldn't be able to make her weekly weight goals. (Don't expect them to have space available when you need it; many have as few as 6-10 beds, so openings are sporadic and most facilities have wait lists.) To our surprise, for five weeks running, she gained enough (though *just* enough) to meet each week's goal. We hadn't been able to anticipate how this would come back to bite us, as things were to unfold.

Toward the end of the sixth week, we received a frantic call from her, pleading for an extra week prior to getting weighed. We knew what this meant: She knew she wasn't going to make that week's goal. Not knowing how to respond, we called the doctor, who insisted we tell her to keep her appointment and who further advised us to start the process of admitting her back into residential. We were devastated. We knew how hard she had worked to gain what she had to for each of the preceding five weeks. Achieving these weight goals might seem relatively simple for those of us without an eating disorder, but for someone struggling with anorexia, this is a monumental fight—every day, all day, with the ED "voice" like a relentless demon inside her head. How she accomplished this, on her own, we'll never fully understand.

By now we are profoundly distressed and confused about what to do. The doctor confirmed by phone that she had not made her goal, insisting that we need stand firm and demand her reentry into residential. But the start of the academic quarter was only two weeks away, she had made so much progress, and she was *so close* to her goal. It would have been one thing if she hadn't met her goals the first couple weeks of the new contract. But with all she had worked so hard to achieve, sending her back—just because we had a contract—felt wrong. It would not only dismiss the massive effort she had put in, it would make us hypocritical. After all, we were asking her ultimately to abandon the "black and white" thinking that characterized much of the mess she was in. Had we stuck to the contract at this point, after she'd made such progress on her own—it would have been *us* mired in " black and white" thinking. She would never forgive us for sending her back to "prison" merely because she'd had "one bad week." We tried putting ourselves in her shoes, and imagined her completely giving up the desire to fight the eating disorder. How could we do that to her, when she'd come so far?

We should not have been surprised, when speaking to the nutritionist and therapist, that *the doctor had not discussed this latest development with other members of team*. They were shocked to learn from us that the doctor had decreed the return to residential. And they adamantly disagreed with the doctor's decision! This caused immense anguish for our daughter and for us—dark days, indeed—which might have been avoided had they coordinated among themselves and then talked with us so that we could all be on "the same page" before communicating the dreaded decision to our daughter.

But at that point, bolstered by the opinions we shared with the rest of the team (other than the doctor), we told our daughter that we were NOT going to send her back to residential because she had done so well up to this last week. Furthermore, we said we would be backing off from our involvement with the treatment team, which we had promised to do if and when we felt she was in recovery. We would no longer be asking for weekly updates concerning her weight, and would simply get updates as we felt we needed them, as long as we had access to the team when we had questions.

Not surprisingly, things went from bad to worse. The doctor, who was understandably angry with us for going against her decree, played the trump card on us. She *advised our daughter to tear up the releases we had worked so hard to get her to sign,* and then announced that she was cutting off communication with us (she would let us know only if our daughter's condition reached the danger point). The doctor apparently had determined that such a "parentectomy" (which is what it is called when parents are excluded from the treatment team) was necessary to preserve our daughter's privacy and autonomy, allowing her to "choose" to eat in order to truly recover. Why is it that the Maudsley approach sees the parents as the most vital part of the team, yet this doctor now regarded *us* as the problem?

Eventually, we negotiated with the doctor for a monthly communication, but in spite of her agreeing to it, we never received one. We spent hours with our own therapist (whom we were able to find after another lengthy argument with the insurance agency to get a single case agreement, so we could find a professional who could help parents dealing with adult children with eating disorders) devising communications with the daughter's team so that we could get some information—any information—about our daughter's condition, as well as about ongoing treatment strategies—to no avail. The doctor's collusion with our daughter's illness (by cutting us out of the treatment process) was the worst loophole yet. She may have been trying to appeal to our daughter's fledgling sense of independence, in the hopes that gaining trust and establishing a therapeutic alliance would cause our daughter to follow her advice. But all we could see was our daughter suffering—withdrawn, defensive, and angry, and continuing to lose weight. We were infuriated at the doctor who, it seemed, had improperly overstepped the bounds of her professional expertise, and was acting as if she were a therapist. This entire situation rendered us completely impotent in saving our child. That late autumn, when we were still being excluded from communication with the team, our daughter came home for the Thanksgiving break. We were glad to have her home—eating disorders thrive on isolation, after all—but we were unnerved and frightened by how she appeared, and how she behaved around food and eating. She didn't want to be watched, she got upset when we even *offered* to purchase food she might eat, much less actually cook anything for her. So we left her alone in the kitchen to make her own snacks and meals. We felt very conflicted about avoiding all talk of food—which felt enabling, but as we have since learned, expressing feelings or concerns directly during certain stages of this illness, could make things much worse. Another Catch-22. It made for an intense holiday, but our primary focus was on having the visit be pleasant enough that she would want to come home for the much longer Christmas vacation one month later. We couldn't bear the possibility of her being alone with her illness over the holidays.

After she'd gone back to school, she called to suggest that we take a trip together over Christmas vacation. Knowing how problematic it was for her socially in our hometown, we wanted to try to accommodate her request. If she could visit relatives on the east coast (who had become alienated when her illness took root), plus visit a university there she was considering for graduate school, it might be a good trip. Some part of her wanted to try to normalize her relationships with those relatives, and maybe having grad school to look forward to would remind her why she had to keep fighting this illness. Even if it *was* only to avoid the toxic social environment at home, it seemed worth doing. Perhaps she was trying to take care of herself emotionally. A positive sign, if so. By now, we were desperate for anything that might give her (and us) the hope and strength to soldier on.
But, how would we pay for that when the expenses for her treatment were killing us? Fortunately, a close friend of the family offered up some frequent flyer miles, and a cousin offered up a place to stay there.

Knowing she wasn't thriving, though, and having witnessed her weight loss over Thanksgiving, we feared she might not be well enough to travel, and worried about her being in the cold winter weather. We wanted to talk to the doctor to find out if it was safe for her to travel. If, for example, the doctor was thinking—or perhaps had initiated conversations with her about the need to re-enter residential treatment—then planning for a trip (the costs for which we couldn't recover if the trip was cancelled) wouldn't make sense. So, in spite of the doctor's refusal to initiate contact with us or respond to our questions about her treatment rationale, we needed an answer to this question. This issue involved other people's money and generosity that we couldn't treat lightly. So we sent the doctor an email asking if it was safe for our daughter to travel and saying that, if she felt a return to residential (or hospitalization) might be likely soon, then we'd have to say no to the trip idea. We asked the doctor to not share our questions with our daughter (as we didn't want to get her hopes up about the trip, or discourage her with our concerns about a potential return to residential).

Whereupon, the doctor did something unimaginable. She responded, saying our daughter could travel (but withheld any indication of her current assessment or concerns for the future), and copied our daughter on her response and *our letter*! This seemed a blatant collusion with the eating disorder as the doctor was clearly more invested in siding with our daughter's wishes to shut us out than in ensuring her safety. Perhaps she reasoned that this would prove to our daughter that she was on her side (against us), in the hopes that it would further align her with the doctor, causing her to heed her advice? Overstepping her role as a physician in order to dabble in an ill-advised psychotherapeutic alliance, the doctor proved no match for the strength of this illness. From our perspective, it had clouded her medical judgment.

When we got past the major upset this caused, we ended up arranging the trip. It went very badly. Our daughter's food restriction was worse than ever; watching this and knowing she believed she was eating enough was beyond heartbreaking. Such discrepancy between reality and the victim's perception of reality is, we now know, a hallmark of anorexia's cognitive distortion. And in many other mental illnesses, that discrepancy might simply be bizarre; in this life-threatening disorder, it was truly terrifying. Everyone on the trip was uncomfortable. Even asking something as simple as "How are you?" elicited a tirade in response. None of this made sense. When at first she insisted that our choice of a restaurant *not* be based on what we thought she might need or like, she subsequently freaked out if she didn't like the place that was chosen. An offer to buy her something that was on her "safe foods" list—thinking something was better than nothing—met with a defiant refusal, every time. She was so upset that she couldn't even drink plain tea at one restaurant (though tea had long been a favorite beverage). We couldn't see any way out of this house of horrors. Why couldn't the doctor see how badly she was failing at the outpatient level of care, when it was painfully obvious to everyone else?

Returning home, we knew she'd lost even more weight on that trip. We were certain the doctor would call us after our daughter's first post-vacation check-up. Surely a return to residential treatment was the next step. But, no call came that week. No call the following week, or the week after that. Finally, we heard from the doctor: "I told you I'd alert you if your daughter became medically unstable, which she is. It is medical malpractice if I continue to see her. She is not safe being at school anymore, and she needs residential care. You have to pull out the big guns and withdraw financial support (from school) because she's so stubborn she won't go otherwise." But, once again, there had been no discussion—much less agreement— among the treatment team. We soon learned that our daughter's therapist disagreed with the doctor's decision, telling us she thought considerable progress had been made in their sessions, and that our daughter's finding things to enjoy about life would help her *decide to eat*. This is a very simplistic concept known as the "feedback loop," which is not at all effective in more acute stages of the illness.

Here we were, yet again, with another loophole created by the treatment team not communicating with each other, deciding whose decision would prevail, and by not presenting a united front. We were certain at this point that our daughter needed nothing short of residential treatment again, and disagreed strongly with the therapist for thinking that her weekly therapy sessions could possibly be enough to get her to eat, especially when the physical evidence of her illness was getting worse, her restriction and rigidity around food was worse, and her thought process around food and family continued to have devolved so greatly. She needed all the support she could get around eating, and enough time in a supportive setting in order to challenge and overcome the forces within her mind that were preventing her from being able to eat properly several times a day.

Worst still, we could not reach the nutritionist. She was out of town and had her phone turned off! She simply disappeared from the team, in spite of knowing our daughter was heading toward crisis and in spite of having promised she would never let our daughter "fall through the cracks." She never surfaced during or after this critical stage!!!!

Finally, the therapist said she'd go along with the doctor's recommendation, but at that point the doctor lost her resolve and told our daughter that she should go to *either* residential or PH – neither of which our daughter was interested in considering – or she would entertain any other idea she could come up with to get better care whilst staying in school! We were furious! When we asked why she was allowing our daughter to come up with a proposal to stay in school, when she specifically told us she was unsafe doing so, the doctor told us not to worry: She had no intention of agreeing to any such proposal (because she didn't believe a reasonable one could be made); rather she felt this was important in allowing our daughter some "say" in the matter. Why raise her hopes and confuse the issue, when she knew she wasn't going to allow it? We were furious. We felt it was cruel to string her along, to give her such false hope.

Nonetheless, we had to act. We had very little time remaining to attack this problem; it was imperative that we arrange for the level of treatment the doctor had said was called for, even though she'd back off from insisting on it. It was up to us to close this loophole. We couldn't force our daughter to go to residential because she over 18. We could have told her we wouldn't pay for her schooling if she didn't go, but we really didn't want to have to use that strategy because we knew that amounted to blackmail in her mind. (And who could argue it wasn't?) We also didn't want her wasting all her energy being angry at us for that, when she needed to focus everything on her recovery.

So, we asked the doctor if she intended to inform the dean of students that our daughter wasn't medically safe continuing on as a student, as she said was the case. She refused to do this because of her interpretation of the HIPAA laws! Our therapist went so far as to call her therapist to argue that they should call the dean of students: that this case is no different that if they had a suicidal patient who was refusing treatment, that they would have a moral and ethical obligation to call the parents and tell them to scoop up their child and bring him or her home. But, fearing a lawsuit (from whom? our ill daughter??) neither the doctor nor the therapist would budge.

So *we* called the dean of students and asked what the school would do in a case like this. The dean made it clear that if a student knowingly refused to follow a physician's orders in a potentially life-threatening situation, the school would not be able, legally, to allow such a student to continue attending classes, and that return to school would only be allowed once the treating physician said the student was healthy enough to return. The same, she said, applied here. We presumed she took this seriously because she didn't want a lawsuit on her hands, should our daughter die. All this remained unspoken.

Our daughter was infuriated when she realized that the dean had eliminated the loophole, and that her only choice was to leave school to pursue treatment. Once she came to terms with this, we still had to get her to choose residential, now that the doctor had waffled and offered her a choice. We had found a new treatment facility near our home; their policy would allow her to continue taking two of her college courses—which we knew would be a major selling point to our daughter. We were also more savvy this time around, and got this facility to agree that any subsequent discharge plan would *require* (1) a step-down to PHP/IOP before returning to school; (2) no returning to school in the spring, regardless (as we knew it would not have been enough time for her reach a healthy weight; and (3) found out what they believed a healthy weight would be and then got assurances that they wouldn't allow her out until she reached that goal. We weren't taking any chances that the treatment center would allow her to leave prematurely, like before. We did not want to create a cycle of hell scenario for her that we have heard so many others have had to traverse with this illness: insufficient treatment in residential, premature discharge, only to relapse and have to continue cycling back into residential or inpatient or worse, time and time again.

Knowing how upset she was at having to leave school mid-quarter, and not wanting to throw away all the hard work she'd done to that point, we went to bat for her to get her what she wanted so she would choose residential. Initially the doctor balked at allowing her to continue her studies (especially without being able to attend classes!), saying it would interfere with the difficult work of recovery. We worked hard to convince the doctor that the residential treatment center staff could monitor the situation and decide if schoolwork was getting in the way; that it would allow her to stay connected to what was critical to her self-esteem; and that it would serve as a daily reminder of what she needed to keep fighting for. Further, that it would allow the treatment team to see the level of perfection that she held herself to, as this trait was connected to her anorexia: the associated compulsivity and perfectionism that had developed in her work habits was either was a causal factor in her anorexia, or was heightened as a result of the anorexia: cause, or effect, or underlying personality trait; in any case, it would be good for the treatment team to assess, we argued.

First we had to convince her therapist to help persuade the doctor of the soundness of our idea. The doctor eventually capitulated, though reluctantly. Then, unexpectedly, the college dean rejected the idea! After much wrangling and pleading, the dean came to see the logic in our argument, and allowed our daughter to continue taking those classes (provided the two professors in question approved the plan, which they did).

Finally, our daughter entered her second residential treatment program. She worked incredibly hard there under the guidance of an excellent staff therapist, but it still remains something of a mystery to us why, this time, she seemed to embrace recovery. We experienced gratifying (though gradual) changes in her demeanor toward us, and we had conversations with her in family therapy that we never thought we'd be able to have. At times, it felt like we were witnessing a phoenix rising from the ashes...some sort of miracle seemed to be taking place, but it is still taking time to shed the doubt and fear we have come to clothe ourselves in.

Following her discharge from residential this time, she entered a PHP/IOP program. Even there, they created loopholes that allowed her to relapse. We agreed to the facility where our daughter had interviewed based on, among other things, their promotion of single-family psychotherapy as an integral part of treatment. What we found out, too late, was that they don't offer that unless 1) the patient asks for it and 2) the patient is willing to *sacrifice her once-weekly individual therapy appointment* to make time for the family sessions. In her case, she wouldn't ask for it (we knew she'd feel it would undermine her attempt to "do this on her own," though we were fairly sure that underlying this was her ED voice wanting to keep us at a safe distance). Most of all, we did not want to shortchange her individual therapy (which we already felt was less than she needed). As a result, we had no opportunity to give the staff our perspective on how she was doing at home. We were seeing increased restriction, but they were giving her increased freedom. With no way to provide vital observations, we were again being marginalized. They only took in the information our daughter presented for the several hours per day she was at the treatment center. As a result, they let her out prematurely. Not surprisingly, she began relapsing the moment she got out! Back at school, she proceeded to lose as much weight in three weeks as she had the first few weeks of her initial weight loss. Months of progress were undone.

To make matters worse, her treatment team back in the college town—the therapist she had been seeing before her stint in residential, plus a new nutritionist and physician—were not in communication at all. Eventually we were able to learn that our daughter had not even been asked to sign a release so her own therapist could communicate with her physician and nutritionist! Her therapist rationalized that this involved an "attachment issue" and that our daughter should take the lead in suggesting any releases be signed. It's one thing for a therapist to allow this of a young adult dealing with attachment and independence issues, but with an exceptionally smart and stubborn young woman struggling with anorexia and its attendant *cognitive distortions*? A therapist who defers to an anorexic patient to take the initiative in giving permission to establish communications with the team is colluding with the illness and creating another enormous loophole.

So, what are the takeaways from this account of our experience?

- First, when you establish a team of professionals, <u>before</u> your child gets into treatment, it's essential to find out what the mechanism is for communicating among the team: who is going to communicate with the family, how often you can expect to hear from them, and by what means? Obtain agreement around protocol, as well—e.g., if you have a question for one member of the team, make sure it's OK to "cc" others (if it's by email) so that everyone stays in the loop and hears the same information exchanged.

- It is critical to determine whose decision will rule in the event of disagreements among the team. For starters, have everyone on the team understand that you—as parents—aren't willing to tolerate loopholes created by the communication of differing opinions. (The ED will capitalize on these, in a heartbeat!) Our non-professional opinion is that in case of lack of consensus about a course of action, the ED-specialist physician (assuming the physician is truly versed in EDs) should have the final say, primarily because the doctor has the hard data about the medical complications caused by the disorder. Having clarity on this point, in advance, among all members of the team will help avoid unnecessary aggravation and lost opportunities to make progress in recovery.

- Make sure that the team will consider parents—who are, after all, the presumed experts in *knowing their child*—an integral part of the team. By having the parental role marginalized at a time when the child (even an adult child) is in the grips of this illness, is setting up a dangerous loophole the eating disorder will walk right through. All loopholes lead to the hidden "slippery slope" that all ED families and treatment teams alike have experienced, often with tragic results.

CHAPTER 6: HIPAA LAWS AND CONSERVATORSHIP/ GUARDIANSHIP

HIPAA Laws

If your child is 18 or older, or about to turn 18 in the near future, you should understand that your efforts to battle anorexia will likely be stymied by HIPAA privacy laws. If your child's illness is severe, and she or he is in denial of the problem, or doesn't want to get better, she holds the trump card. With privacy laws on her side, she doesn't have to sign releases in order for you to be able to communicate with the treatment team. You will need to develop a strategy to outwit the law.

HIPAA is the Health Insurance Portability and Accountability Act of 1996. It decrees that for patients over 18, doctors or mental health providers must have a signed "release of information authorization" before they can share any information with parents, other professionals and treatment facilities, or other individuals—and only then as specified by the patient. With an **egosyntonic** disorder such as anorexia—in which the behaviors and feelings are perceived by the victim as *harmonious with her identity* and aligned with her needs and values—having to share information with parents and others becomes a threat to her ego-protection paradigm. And yes, the law protects the patient's privacy rights, even when the parents are paying for treatment!

This becomes extremely problematic when parents need to communicate with the treatment team to evaluate the caregivers' qualifications; to understand the treatment strategy; and to be aware of ongoing assessments, goals and contingency plans (which may need the parents' buy-in, to succeed). Keeping parents out of the communication loop also prevents consideration of vital information from those who often intimately observe anorexic behaviors (including food restriction) outside the treatment setting, which is often at odds with data being provided by the patient.

Eating disorders survive on deceit and manipulation: They will do and say *anything* to throw parents, well-meaning friends, and treatment providers off-track; they are masters at appearing "fine" on the surface. Even medical exams and lab tests can deceive: Blood work of an anorexic may show up in the normal range (due to the medical phenomenon of homeostasis, the mechanism for which is not fully understood); sometimes scales won't register weight loss because of tricks some patients use (i.e., "water loading" prior to a weigh-in, or hiding weights in the hair or other orifices); a low heart rate can be disguised by consuming caffeine or other stimulants prior to exam. Some doctors are savvy enough to make these patients do jumping jacks before they step on the scales, to dislodge any hidden weights, but others don't even ask the patient to disrobe (what girl doesn't know how to use clothing to mask weight gain or loss?).

In any case, it only makes sense that the team should want to get a complete picture of what is really going on—throughout the complete course of evaluation, treatment and recovery—and HIPAA laws systematically exclude those who could provide such information.

When our daughter was a high school senior, before she became ill, we happened to attend a school event in which parents shared their experiences of the college application process and the student's first year away from home. One parent said the most important piece of advice she could give was to make sure to have the child sign an "Authorization to Release Information" form (available on college websites). She hadn't known to do this, and when her son was involved in a serious bike accident, the hospital staff would not disclose how the boy was doing or what they intended to do to him. Furthermore, his accident had rendered him incapable of signing anything (he was already on the operating table). Frantic and unable to get any information, they flew across the country and arrived at the hospital to take charge of their son's life. Heeding that mother's advice, we made sure to take care of this over the summer before our daughter headed to school, having no clue of course about the impending disaster looming on our horizon.

Even so, when she spiraled out of control with anorexia and we insisted on setting up a treatment team as a condition for her going back to school, she suddenly remembered having signed the release the previous summer. During our meeting with the school's student-health liaison, our daughter demanded the form be rewritten in a way calculated to keep us at bay about her anorexia. Confronted with the conflicting desire to show her we respected her need for autonomy while also knowing we wanted access to her treatment team, we compromised on what we thought would give us a minimal amount of general information. We had no way of knowing then that we should have specified in detail how our contact with the team would work (e.g., whether we could talk to the team members, whether or how often they could communicate with us, what kind of information they could provide, and so much more that became apparent over time).

In the month following that meeting, we had the chance to observe our daughter (at an "away" sporting event). Her behavior was so bizarre and her food-restricting so extreme that we felt it essential to share our observations and concerns in a letter to her therapist and the school physician (especially given the university's moral and legal obligation to restrict her participation in intercollegiate sports in her deteriorating condition).

The doctor's response was both appalling and predictable: She cited HIPAA privacy concerns, refused to lend our concerns any credibility, and dismissed us with a reminder about how important autonomy is to every 18-year-old. We were livid. Moreover, we were distressed to realize that our daughter's life was not in capable hands. One didn't have to be a doctor to see how ill she was, but the medical director of a college health center who lacks the qualifications to accurately assess eating disorders is a truly terrifying notion. (To her credit, over the next few months she apologized to us, saying she too had been "outsmarted" by our daughter's illness, which only shows how devious anorexia can be when manifest in someone who is both charming and highly intelligent.) But, at the time, we were furious at being patronized and worried sick about our child and her rapid decline.

We decided we had to stare down this monster or forever be at its mercy. We emailed our daughter an ultimatum: Either give us full access to the team (which, being 18, she had no legal obligation to do) or we would withdraw financial support for her to continue at college (which we were under no legal obligation to provide!). After considerable wrangling (including being accused of "blackmail" by holding the school funding over her head), we got the releases signed, but before long her condition deteriorated to the point that she had to be placed in residential care.

Many professionals in this field advise parents to use any tool at their disposal to force the appropriate level of care. Blackmail or not, we felt we had no choice but to withdraw funding if we were going to have any hope of saving her life. But for sufferers of anorexia who may no longer be dependent on parents for school, housing or living expenses, what leverage do these loved ones have?

It seems a daunting task to advocate for an amendment to the HIPAA laws, though a worthwhile task for those who are willing and able to spend their energies in such an endeavor.

Conservatorship/Guardianship

If your child is an independent adult, yet is unable to make rational decisions about her health (such as managing the essential act of taking in adequate nourishment to ensure survival), you can consult an attorney who specializes in conservatorship or guardianship (states use different terms, but they mean the same thing). The power of the state to put someone in charge of another adult's welfare is a tricky business even under optimum conditions. With eating disorders, it is exceedingly difficult for a variety of reasons—but not impossible.

We are not attorneys and will not attempt a comprehensive treatment of the topic here. Suffice to say that we have heard that it is incredibly difficult to get a judge to rule in favor of families trying to help a child with an eating disorder. Even though anorexia is classified as a mental illness and even though it is possible to obtain a conservatorship for those suffering with debilitating mental illness, the legal system is not yet educated to the realities and complexities of eating disorders. To take just one aspect: Severely distorted cognitive functioning in some areas (due to malnutrition, in this case) is not the same as psychosis, so a person who exhibits reasonable decision-making capability in other areas of her life will not have a hard time convincing most judges to protect her right to self-determination—even when everyone around her can see she is slowly starving herself to death. Carrie Arnold, the author of a few books on anorexia, introduces an article in her blog (ed-bites.blogspot.com) written by Professor Arthur Caplan, University of Pennsylvania, called "Denying Autonomy in Order to Create It: The Paradox of Forcing Treatment Upon Addicts." The article explores the conundrum of addiction, self-determination, competence, and autonomy. Addiction involves a loss of control, power and the ability to manage; caught up in behavioral compulsion, the addict is not able to make autonomous decisions. Competence, by itself, is not sufficient for autonomy, because autonomy requires freedom from coercion. Therefore, if compulsory treatment (such as by granting conservatorship) can remove the coercion of causing powerlessness and loss of control by denying autonomy to a person with an eating disorder or an addiction, it may actually free her up to *be* autonomous, quite capable of self-determination. Carrie points out that most people with eating disorders resist having their right to self-determination taken away, but points to a study in which many clients acknowledged, at some point during their treatment, that the treatment was necessary.

In our case, we couldn't understand how our child could be so oblivious to her deteriorating health. Part of the smokescreen she used to convince us she was OK and still in control was her academic performance. She got the highest grades possible in every subject (not just in her major), even when she was most severely afflicted with the illness. How could this be, when she could barely function in so many other aspects of her life? We posed this question to a leading researcher in the field, and while he couldn't answer definitively, he explained that the current belief among many experts is that the extreme focus and the drive for perfection—such as would cause a student to be satisfied with nothing less than the maximum possible scores— is *part of the psychopathology* of this illness. It is also known that as the illness becomes chronic and severe over time, cognitive functioning in areas unrelated to food also becomes compromised. But by the time this occurs, it could be too late. By this time, they may have either died, or become so entrenched in the illness to have rendered full recovery all that much more difficult.

One can't blame judges who have a limited understanding of the mechanisms of this disease; after all, even many doctors, nutritionists and therapists have been slow to fully comprehend this insidious illness (to say nothing of agreeing on the most effective treatment strategies). If we had pursued conservatorship, our daughter could easily have demonstrated her mental acuity (her charm and cleverness were well-established long before anorexia set in). And unless the judge happened to be well-versed in the mysterious way in which anorexia renders patients incapable of making rational decisions about their health (yet so capable in other areas), any legal effort to take control of her life seemed doomed to fail, at least in California. The one glimmer of hope we heard was that judges in Oregon are more progressive than most in California, and that caretakers at a certain clinic in that state may help in the filing and serving of conservatorship documents.

In any case, it is worth investigating if conservatorship is an option. Otherwise, if you have an adult child who is ill, you will need to get very creative in trying to persuade her that she needs help. You can consider letting him or her know that you will not provide financial support unless they enter treatment but these are very difficult choices and even harder to make when their illness becomes chronic and they become so entrenched in it that they can't envision or figure out how to create a life without it. Tough love doesn't necessarily work with an illness like this. You can't just put your ill child out on the street and expect her to suddenly understand that you mean business, and expect acquiesce to enter treatment. All the more reason that taking decisive action early on in the illness provides better chances for recovery.

College Tuition Refund Policy

Finally, we understand that some colleges and universities offer a tuition-refund policy. Purchasing this policy may help alleviate the added stress of losing tuition in case your child needs to take a medical leave. Indeed, given the lack of medical insurance coverage for residential treatment of eating disorders, you may need those tuition funds to pay to save your child's life. What are the takeaways from this chapter?

- If your child is ill when they are under 18 and living at home, pull out all the stops and do everything to insist on recovery. You have all your parent controls available to you at this stage.

- If your child is not sick when he or she goes to college, or has been ill and is in a stage of recovery such that you are willing to chance sending him or her off to college, get releases filled out and signed in advance (and keep a copy in your files). That way, regardless of whether your child becomes afflicted with an eating disorder—or suffers a relapse of a previously existing eating disorder—you will have established the legal right to be part of your child's team. And if he or she gets hospitalized for some other reason, you can show the form to the hospital or other treatment professionals so that they can let you know what is going on.

- It is worth considering telling your child that a condition of their going away to school is that you will have releases. We wish we had known enough before our daughter left for school to tell her that those were our conditions for supporting her during her college years. Hindsight is, indeed 20-20.

- We highly recommend that you consult a lawyer who can help you navigate the complex arena of conservatorship, and gather information on what is possible in your state.

CHAPTER SEVEN: INSURANCE COVERAGE

Insurance coverage in the United States is indeed a complicated topic, and the cost for all forms of treatment for eating disorders is extremely high. Many residential treatment centers cost up to $1300 or more per day, and require a deposit (that you are refunded, if all goes well) as well a payment upfront for the first few treatment days. Some PHPs bill at $900 per day, with half-day IOP programs charging $600 per day. The nutritionist at the IOP was charging us $450 for 3-hour segments, and she claimed she spent far many more sessions with her than we knew our daughter was attending. These amounts are only what we know of from our own experience. The point here is that treatment is enormously expensive and having insurance is essential for most parents to afford the proper level of care. We also know that having insurance doesn't mean it will cover all the related expenses. Below is some information we hope will be helpful.

Dependents Can Be Insured Until Their 27th Birthday. The first thing to keep in mind regarding insurance for treatment of eating disorders is that under the Affordable Care Act (effective March 2010), if an insurance plan offers dependent coverage, they must make the coverage available to adult children up through age 26. Young adults are eligible for coverage even if they are married, not living with you, attending school, not financially dependent on you, or even if they are eligible to enroll in their employer's plan. There are some exceptions, however. For employer plans that were in existence prior to the date of enactment, young adult children can qualify for dependent coverage only if they are not eligible for an employment-based health insurance plan until 2014, but beginning in 2014, they can choose to stay on their parent's health plan until age 26, even if they are eligible for their own employer-sponsored insurance plan. Plans are required to provide a 30-day enrollment period prior to the plan's next "policy year" for you to enroll your child. You would need to speak with your employer or research further to find out if it is possible to enroll your child outside of this enrollment period.

University Health Insurance. If you are a parent of a child heading for college, you will be faced with the decision of whether to have your child also enroll in the school's health insurance policy, assuming the school offers one. In our case, enrollment in the university health insurance plan was automatic, although we were given the option to file a waiver to opt out of that additional coverage. At first, being budget-conscious, we considered filing a waiver. After all, we had our family insurance, and it would save us $1200 per year in fees. We ultimately decided against filing a waiver, but only for the sake of convenience. The Student Health Service at her school is located right on campus, and it's free for those with university insurance. If she couldn't utilize that for free (which she could if she enrolled in student insurance), we would either have to pay each time she went, or she would have hassle with finding Blue Shield network providers off campus, which is a hassle as well as a commute. So, we bit the bullet and decided to pay for it.

Best decision we ever made, though of course we didn't know it at the time, nor did we do it with any sense of why it was going to be so important for us. What we found out, in a moment of extreme anxiety and concern over our daughter's health, was that our own insurance, Blue Shield, didn't cover residential treatment at all. With residential treatment facility fees at $1,450 per day, although a bit less thanks to their provider discount it), if we hadn't had the additional student insurance for her, we would have been hit with a $70,000 bill – and that's just for the 9 weeks she stayed. Had she not been let out prematurely, that fee could easily have doubled. While we still had to come up with a sizeable "out-of-pocket" fee, it was far better than what could easily have been our plight – possibly having to sell our house???? Fortunately, the school's insurance policy did cover it (though that was granted as a "single case agreement" – and we didn't know that she would qualify for coverage until late in the afternoon of the day before her being admitted!), although we had a significant out-of-pocket payment. Given this experience, we would highly recommend paying for school insurance policy, especially if you have an adolescent at home who has had an eating disorder who has college in his or her future.

Problems with Insurance Company's Covering Patients with Eating Disorders. Dealing with insurance companies has, at times, added much anxiety for us, particularly difficult because it occurs often when patients are in the midst of a transition in care when anxiety levels are already extreme as a result of the illness.

Finding Expert Providers on Insurance Panels/Single Case Agreements. One problem we have encountered is finding providers who are on their insurance panels.

Each time we have had to search for treatment providers, we have had to find those who are "in network" providers. It was very difficult finding those "in network" for our daughter. Fortunately, by having two insurance policies to work with, we were able to work with two lists. Unfortunately, however, in both cases, there were only a few who understood or were expert in anorexia. We couldn't afford to consider other providers who are not in network. The only exception is if you can prove to the insurance company that they don't have an expert in a particular field. For example, there were many psychotherapists who listed themselves as expert in eating disorders on the panel, but none of the psychiatrists in her school town who were on either panel had expertise with anorexia. We had to call each psychiatrist on the list provided by the insurance company to ascertain that ourselves, then call the insurance company to tell them what the providers told us; then the insurance agent had to call those providers to verify that what we said was true. It was only then that we were able to get them to approve what is called a "single case agreement" (SCA) – in effect, a special contract that the insurance makes with a provider not on their panel. And this can only happen if the provider is willing to negotiate a rate with the insurance company that may be lower than their normal rates, and be willing to comply with the oversight and paperwork required by the insurance company. Many providers are not interested in having their clinical judgments being overridden by someone at an insurance company who has never even met their patients.

We also felt it was necessary for us, as parents, to find a therapist so that we could have an expert help us sort through our own issues pertaining to our daughter's anorexia, and get guidance by an expert in how to communicate with someone afflicted as well as with her treatment team. We were told by our daughter's team that we needed to "back off" and not express our concerns to our daughter, as she couldn't deal with our anxieties on top of her own. We often felt conflicted with this because we felt that not confronting things enabled her to carry on with eating disordered behaviors. We needed a lot of help figuring out how to communicate with her and with her team, and at times we needed our therapist to be a liaison with her team so that our concerns could be conveyed when the team wouldn't listen to us, but also so we could obtain information that they would not provide directly to us.

Finding our own therapist who was (a) knowledgeable about eating disorders, (b) had experience working directly with anorexic patients, and (c) had worked with parents dealing with *adult* children with anorexia, presented a major challenge.

Upon our request, Blue Shield provided us with a list of therapists in located nearby; the list had been generated by sorting on the key words "eating disorders." It didn't take us long to figure out that when therapists join insurance panels, they merely tick off a variety of boxes next to the ailments they say they can treat. This does NOT mean they are qualified ED experts, or have worked with a minimum number of ED patients, or have gone through specialized training. It may simply include a normative desire to work with such clients. We didn't know this up front, but as we spoke with each therapist and asked whether he or she had worked with parents of adult anorexics, it turned out many never had. One therapist we called admitted it had been a dozen years since she'd worked with an ED client; another said her expertise was in helping women fulfill their life desires; still another decreed—over the phone, in the first three minutes of our conversation—that Lyn's problem was that she had overfed our daughter and was a controlling mom! In short, providers can tick off any subspecialty they like; this allows them to cast a wide net in search of clients, but it creates enormous risks for unwary and unquestioning ED clients.

This was a very frustrating endeavor. It required many calls, taking notes on when I had spoken to whom, then calling the insurance company back to report that none of the options they gave me were appropriate. Then, waiting for days until the insurance company could report back that they had verified what I told them by calling the providers back. When we asked for a single case agreement to cover a therapist we had found who was not on their panel, they then widened their geographical search to include therapists who were 40 or more miles away. I had to argue that there was no way the insurance agency could find it acceptable for us to not only have to take time off of work, but then spend an extra hour and a half or more just in the commute to and from appointments.

Meanwhile, we were in mid-crisis, floundering on the proverbial creek without a paddle. Trying to manage this, while dealing with our daughter and her treatment providers, etc. meant taking significant time off of work, which added to our financial worries as well. Finding our own ED therapist was, of course, secondary to ensuring our daughter's safety. So we put the search on hold until the summer, when I wasn't working and would theoretically have more time. Once we restarted the search, I had to call more than 30 providers on Blue Shield's list before they granted us a single case agreement for an out-of-network therapist.

As difficult as it can be to find treatment providers on insurance panels, keep in mind that you can request a single case agreement if you can prove that there are no experts on their in-network list of providers. We have met many parents along the way who didn't know this option existed.

Insurance Companies Denying Coverage of Treatment

First, Blue Shield (at the time) didn't even cover residential treatment – it is blatantly written so in their policy (although this may change, thanks to a recent ruling which we'll explain below), and it was unclear whether her school insurance would, as their policy didn't even address it. Fortunately, the school insurance did cover it, though we didn't get final word until the day before she was admitted. We had a hefty "out-of-pocket" – which had to be paid up front before the insurance kicked in, but we were fortunate because it was a lot lower than the amount we would have had to pay. (For 9 weeks, it cost $70,000, and that was with a 20% provider discount, so had we not had insurance, we would have had to pay $84,000 - plus we were looking at double that amount if she stayed for the full 4 months her physician indicated would be necessary to properly launch her recovery. So we were really fortunate to have not opted out of that school insurance.

Secondly, when she left residential care prematurely, and was in a Level 2 outpatient setting, we suddenly received a letter from Blue Shield saying that they had decided to deny her coverage. We received this letter the day their coverage ended! According to Blue Shield, she "no longer meets the criteria" for coverage in intensive outpatient; she "no longer has symptoms and a history that demonstrates a significant likelihood of deterioration in function or relapse if transitioned to a less intensive level of care;" and – with seemingly contradictory logic – stated that she was being denied because she had "not made measurable and realistic progress."

We were shocked, frantic, running scared. At this point in time, her physician was telling us she needed to go back to residential care (in effect, switch from Level 2 to Level 4 care) because she was failing in outpatient care, both physically and mentally. Her depression and anxiety were at extreme levels; she was not able to eat and was losing weight. Physically, her labs indicated her thyroid function was getting worse, her serum cortisol (which is indicative of her body's stress levels) was increasing, and other markers showed she wasn't consuming enough protein. She was extremely malnourished.

Appealing Insurance Denials.

Not at the time understanding that the other insurance would be the default wallet for our troubles, and worried about how to pay the $10,000-$14,000 per month we were being charged for the IOP treatment, we requested an expedited (3-day) appeal, which was turned down. We then filed a normal appeal. That got denied as well. We then filed an Independent Medical Review (IMR), and fortunately got the denial overturned.

At first, we appealed out of fear about how we would cover these costs. Even though it became clear that the payment defaulted to our secondary insurance (the university insurance), we still felt the need to follow through with the appeal. The university insurance expected a co-pay from us of 20% - which was still beyond our means, but even when the treatment provider promised to waive that 20% for us, we felt a moral obligation to pursue the appeal: We felt Blue Shield should be held accountable for covering these costs. They shouldn't get out of it because they wanted to protect their bottom line, and even go so far as to contradict their own logic in the pursuit of that objective. They shouldn't be allowed to bully people, just because they assume most people won't have the time and energy to fight back. Most importantly, we felt the insurance company should be held accountable for future patients. What if (and surely there will be) in the future, patients struggling with eating disorders only have Blue Shield insurance, and find that they can't get their outpatient treatment covered because the company keeps on being allowed to find ways to deny coverage? Will these patients be forced to withdraw from treatment as a result, only to be allowed to suffer silently alone in their apartments? Too many people suffer without treatment because of insurance denials. We felt it important to hold Blue Shield accountable for these scenarios as well.

To file the appeal, we had to write a letter and address each of the arguments Blue Shield made. We researched the American Psychiatric Association Levels of Care Guidelines, and used that as a basis of rebutting each one of their points, in an effort to show that she clearly met criteria not only for the level of care they were denying but also for a higher level of care. This involved coordinating with the physician and nutritionist, as they needed to contribute written assessments as well.

We were surprised when the appeal was denied, but we didn't stop there. We took it to the state level, requesting an "Independent Medical Review" (IMR), in which physicians who are supposedly expert in the field of eating disorders, but who are not affiliated with the insurance company, review the case. Fortunately, we won the appeal. It didn't end up making a huge difference for us, personally, but Blue Shield was forced to cover those costs, and the other insurance company was reimbursed for the most of the payments they had made.

Fighting insurance companies is not uncommon, where eating disorders are concerned. Many people have fought insurance companies; some have lost, some have won. Every state has different insurance laws, and every policy offers different benefits. We recommend reading Dr. Pamela Carlton's book, Take Charge of Your Child's Eating Disorder, which devotes a chapter to insurance-related issues. Check the resources listed in Chapter 9 of this book, as well, as may have information on how to handle insurance.

Parity Laws
It would be wise to become familiar with the federal Mental Health Parity Act (MHPA), which was signed into law in 1996. Prior to the enactment of this law, most health insurance policies covered mental illnesses at levels far below that for other physical illnesses. This inadequate treatment of mental illnesses is noted to have caused relapse and untold suffering for people with treatable mental illnesses.

The parity law requires insurance companies that offer group plans (with some exceptions) to cover mental health benefits in parity with medical benefits. In order words, the dollar limit allowed for mental health coverage and the lifetime dollar limits on mental health benefits cannot be lower than the limits allowed for medical and surgical benefits. However, each state has different parity laws. In California, the law specifically includes a provision for anorexia and bulimia. To understand what your state offers, check http://takeaction.mentalhealthamerica.net/site/DocServer/Parity_Chart_200 8_1_.pdf?docID=1161. You can also check the Department of Labor website: www.dol.gov/ebsa/newsroom/fsmhparity.html for more information on parity laws. The National Alliance on Mental Illness's website includes a chart that clarifies what each state offers, as well: http://www.nami.org/Content/ContentGroups/Policy/Issues_Spotlights/P arity1/State_Parity_Chart_0709.pdf.

Thanks to these parity laws, the persistence of a mother of a patient with anorexia whose residential treatment was denied by Blue Shield, and the tireless work of her lawyer, Lisa Kantor (at Kantor & Kantor, LLP), on August 26, 2011, the 9th U.S. Circuit Court of Appeals held in *Harlick v. Blue Shield of California*, 2011 DJDAR 13132 that *"health care plans falling within the scope of California's Mental Health Parity Act must provide all medically necessary treatment to the people they insure that suffer from any one of nine specified severe mental illnesses."* The nine specific severe mental illnesses include schizophrenia, schizoaffective disorder, bipolar disorder, major depressive disorders, panic disorder, obsessive-compulsive disorder, pervasive developmental disorder or autism, anorexia nervosa, and bulimia nervosa. Fortunately, in California, these eating disorders are specified in the parity laws.

Jeanene Harlick, the woman whose mother filed the suit, has the same Blue Shield HMO Coverage as we do. In her case, the Blue Shield lawyers tried to argue that since there is no treatment for physical illness equivalent to residential treatment, residential care shouldn't have to be covered under the parity laws. They tried to argue that residential is equivalent to assisted living, which the company doesn't cover for medical illnesses, and therefore shouldn't have to pay on behalf of eating disordered patients. But Lisa Kantor argued successfully that residential care is equivalent to a skilled nursing facility, and therefore Blue Shield should pay in parity with that. Ultimately, the court ruled that, even though Blue Shield's policy excludes residential care facilities, Blue Shield can't exclude residential facilities from coverage as a matter of law, given that treatment was considered medically necessary.

Blue Shield countered with a request for a rehearing, but on June 5, 2012, the United States Court of Appeals for the Ninth Circuit upheld its original decision that the California Mental Health Parity Act requires health plans to provide coverage of "all medically necessary treatment" for "severe mental illnesses" under "the same financial terms as those applied to physical illnesses." In this latest decision, the court held that **health plans in California are obligated to pay for residential treatment for people with eating disorders even if the policy excludes residential treatment.** This is a major victory for people who suffer from eating disorders, yet it remains unclear what impact the decision will have on California's 3.4 million policyholders, or the rest of the nation in which there are an estimated 24 million who suffer from eating disorders, which have the highest fatality rate of any psychiatric disorder.

At the NEDA 2011 Conference in Hollywood, we had the privilege of sitting in a session led by Lisa Kantor. She explained that we should all take note of some basic facts:

- If you have private insurance (i.e., not provided through your employer), it is not necessary to file an appeal before you bring on a lawsuit. In these lawsuits, juries decide outcomes, evidence can be admitted which is not in the insurance company's claims folder, and you can sue for damages above and beyond the cost of insurance and legal fees.

- However, if your insurance is provided by an employer, insurance is operated under the ERISA laws (except if you are in the military or receive insurance from a religious organization). ERISA, The Employee Retirement Income Security Act of 1974, protects the interests of participants and their beneficiaries who depend on benefits from private employee benefit plans. If you have been denied coverage, you are required to file an appeal before you file a lawsuit. In these cases, a judge will rule (so it will depend on the judge), you are unable to sue for more than the cost of treatment and legal feels, and the judge will only admit into evidence that which is in the insurance company claims folder. This means it is essential that, after every conversation you have with an insurance agent you send a letter to them recapping what transpired in the conversation, and send the letter certified and with return receipt.

- You should note that ERISA imposes higher-than-marketplace quality standards on insurers: The plan administrator must discharge its services solely in the interests of the participants and beneficiaries of the plan, and they must provide a full and fair review of claim denials. If you feel you aren't being treated with your interests paramount, you might remind them of this.

- You should be aware that doctors on insurance companies who deny coverage may have stock in the insurance company, so they benefit by denying coverage, as it lowers corporate expenditures. Ask if the doctor has stock options or other vested interests, and what their qualifications are with regard to expertise on eating disorders.

- You can lose the case if you withdraw from treatment in the middle of a review, so it is important to continue with treatment. Apparently, there is federal legislation that is attempting to ensure that insurance continue to cover expenses during the appeals process, but this hasn't been decided yet.

Make sure to work with the providers to see if they can work out a plan to continue with treatment during the appeals process.

- It is also legal to bill for a lower level of care than what is being delivered. So, if an insurance company denies coverage when your child is in residential care, you can ask the facility to charge insurance for the PHP part of the treatment (which could be around $900 per day vs. $1300 or more.) If the treatment providers feel that the patient needs PHP at a minimum, then there is the possibility that an insurance company, such as Blue Shield—which blatantly denies residential treatment coverage—will at least cover a significant portion of the cost, which would allow your child to continue receiving treatment. This is far better than stopping treatment that is considered necessary, especially considering the information in the bullet point above.

- You are entitled to a copy of the claim file before the appeal.

In summary, then, for this chapter:

- Remember that your kids can be on your family insurance policy until their 27th birthday.

- If your child is heading to college, it may be wise to purchase the university insurance, as we happened to. It saved us untold agony because at the time, our family policy didn't cover residential treatment.

- You can ask the insurance company for a "Single Case Agreement" so that they will cover the costs of a provider not in their network. You many need to prove to them that they don't have anyone on their panel who is expert, and this may take a lot of time, but it is an option.

- If you are denied insurance and you choose to appeal, if you obtain your insurance through yours or your spouse's company plan, you will have to file an appeal before you can file a lawsuit.

- If you are not treated with respect by the insurance agents, make sure to remind them that ERISA requires them to consider ONLY your rights as a consumer.

- It is essential to keep good records, and if you have conversations with the insurance companies, make sure to follow up every conversation with a letter reiterating what you understood took place in the conversation, so that it gets in your file. If you have to resort to litigation, if you have insurance through your workplace, appeals are under the HIPPA laws, and judges will only admit into evidence that which is in the insurance company's claim file.

- And, again: Document, document, document!

PART THREE: TOOLS OF THE TRADE

CHAPTER EIGHT: GETTING ORGANIZED

Dealing with a situation like this is overwhelming: Countless phone calls trying to identify or work with treatment professionals, endless emails soliciting advice from experts or just those who've "been there," navigating the esoteric maze of insurance, and so on

It's emotionally exhausting to do all that while adjusting to the changes in your child's appearance and behavior, endlessly discussing how best to deal with all of it—while at the same time holding down a job, and/or taking care of the rest of the family with their own needs as well as their responses to the one with the eating disorder.

Given that parents of adolescents or young adults with eating disorders may also be dealing with the personal challenges of middle age (including simultaneous care of *their* aging parents), our advice is simple: Get and stay as ORGANIZED as possible, because otherwise you'll drown in the complexity, uncertainty, anguish and expense of it all; whether you like it or not, you will become the field general in charge of this multi-layered battle against the eating-disorder forces, and the more organized and strategic and prepared you can be, at every step of the way, the better.

To deal with the morass, I developed the habit of keeping a diary; the time invested in doing so paid huge dividends later, in ways we never could have imagined. Here's a two-entry example:

September 1, 2010

- *Called insurance rep (name, number) at school to find out if Dr. T would be covered on school insurance. Dr. T. not on that plan.*
- *Called Blue Shield (name, number) to ask if Dr. T's on their provider network. She didn't know. Said to check x website.*
- *Checked website. Dr. not on plan.*
- *Called school rep to ask if insurance would issue single case agreement (SCA). She said she'd call back.*
- *Called Dr. T's office. Asked if they'd bill insurance directly if we could get SCA. They said no. But if insurance doesn't cover, they will only charge half.*
- *Texted daughter. No reply.*

September 2, 2010

- *Called Jen at X residential facility (phone #) to see if they have any space upcoming. Not for 3 weeks or more.*
- *Called Jill at Y residential facility to see if they have space. They do, but only if she enters on such-and-such date.*
- *Called daughter's doctor to see what her current thought is about need for residential treatment. She says wait a week.*

This kind of daily documentation not only retained useful information that would otherwise have been forgotten or lost, it has kept us sane! It enabled us to refer back through the muck of the chaos and not have to fumble around trying to recollect or dig up information. Moreover, it has helped us reflect back on complicated, emotionally charged conversations more accurately, especially when family therapy and later recovery steps could be bolstered by what happened and what was said previously.

Secondly, we recommend purchasing two large binders, a few packets of index tabs, and a notebook: one binder for all the miscellaneous paperwork you collect on treatment centers, pages printed from websites, et al., and one for insurance and medical issues. The first binder is useful if you have a running, chronological hard copy log for notes taken at or following support groups, therapy sessions, etc.

In the insurance binder, each index tab could be for the different insurance companies, and for each professional, and as you file each EOB, insurance paper, we recommend you log all expenses in an Excel worksheet.

Finally, per the advice of a prominent attorney who specializes in eating disorder cases, make sure to DOCUMENT each and every conversation you have with insurance companies. We have been told that, as soon as you get off the phone with them, write up notes on your conversation, and send them by certified mail, return receipt, and keep a copy for your file. If you end up in a legal battle with insurance, this documentation will be necessary to have in your file at the insurance company.

It is hard to fathom the additional stress we would have suffered had we not been so organized, from the beginning. If you're not sure how much to save or record, our advice is: EVERYTHING!

CHAPTER NINE: RESOURCES TO KNOW ABOUT

Websites:

Acronym	Organization	Website	Purpose
IAEDP	International Association of Eating Disorder Professionals	www.iaedp.com	The IAEDP provides education, training, and certification to an international multidisciplinary group of healthcare providers who treat the full spectrum of eating disorder problems.
NEDA	National Eating Disorders Association	www.nationaleatingdisorders.com	Treatment referrals, a medical advocacy program, linked to other eating disorder associations and national advocacy.
AED	Academy of Eating Disorders	www.aedweb.org	Professional organization dedicated to leadership in eating disorders research, education, treatment and prevention.
ANAD	National Association of Anorexia Nervosa and Associated Disorders	www.anad.org	A non-profit dedicated to the prevention and alleviation of eating disorders.
EDRS	Eating Disorder Recovery Support, Inc.	www.edrs.net	Awareness, professional education and collaboration, treatment, scholarship for California residents
	Something Fishy	www.something-fishy.org	Pro-recovery website
EDC	Eating Disorders	www.eatingdisor	Advocacy at the federal level

	Coalition	derscoalition.org	
	Anna Westin Foundation	www.annawestin foundation.org	Assists those suffering directly or indirectly from eating disorders; provides education and information designed to prevent the development of anorexia and bulimia.
NIS	Normal In Schools	www.normal-life.org	A national art and education non-profit which teaches about eating disorders, body image and self esteem. NIS founder, Robyn Hussa, produced a very important film, "Speaking Out About ED," which debunks myths, explores treatment options, and calls for better training of the medical community in managing this threatening condition.
The Alliance	The Alliance for Eating Disorders Awareness	www.alliancefor eatingdisorders.c om	A source of community outreach, education, awareness, and prevention of the various eating disorders currently plaguing our nation. Their aim is to share the message that recovery from these disorders is possible, and that individuals should not have to suffer or recover alone.
	Ophelia's Place	www.opheliaspla ce.org	Empowers people to redefine beauty and health, and provides outreach, advocacy and educational services to those impacted by eating disorders, disordered eating and body dissatisfaction. Offers support groups, information on treatment options, workshops, conferences, and a full service café.
	Andrea's Voice Foundation	www.andreasvoic e.org	After their daughter lost her very short battle with bulimia, Doris and Tom Smelter have sought to educate others on this so often misunderstood illness. After they wrote the book, Andrea's Voice, they established this non-profit to continue their work.
	Mentor Connect	www.mentorcon nect-ed.org	The first global eating disorders mentoring community that aims to break through the isolation of eating disorders by connecting members with mentors to share experiences, provide guidance, and help each other through the struggles and triumphs of recovery.

NIMH	National Institute of Mental Health	www.nimh.nih.gov	The mission of NIMH is to transform the understanding and treatment of mental illnesses through basic and clinical research, paving the way for prevention, recovery, and cure.
	Eating Disorder Referral and Information Center	www.edreferral.com	A place to search for treatment and read recent ED articles.
MEDA	Multiservice Eating Disorder Association	www.medainc.org	Dedicated to the prevention and treatment of eating disorders and disordered eating through educational awareness and early detection. A support network and resource for clients, loved ones, clinicians, educators and the general public.
FEAST-ED	Families Empowered and Supporting the Treatment of Eating Disorders	www.feast-ed.org	F.E.A.S.T. is an international organization of and for parents and caregivers to help loved ones recover from eating disorders by providing information and mutual support, promoting evidence-based treatment, and advocating for research and education to reduce the suffering associated with eating disorders.
	Maudsley Parents	www.maudsleyparents.org	Maudsley Parents is a volunteer organization of parents who have helped their children recover from anorexia and bulimia through the use of a family-based treatment known as the Maudsley approach, an evidence-based therapy for eating disorders. They invite everyone to explore their site to learn more about how families can help their kids with eating disorders. Research shows long term outcomes with family-based treatment are promising.
	Training Institute for Child and Adolescent Eating Disorders	http://train2treat4ed.com/certifiedfbttherapists.html	Contact Information for Certified FBT Therapists.
	Eating Disorder Hope	www.eatingdisorderhope.com/	Eating Disorder Hope offers information, treatment options, support groups, information on recovery tools and resources to those suffering, their treatment provides ad

			their loved ones.
	US Library of Medicine, National Institutes of Health Medical Publications Site	www.pubmed.gov	PubMed contains more than 21 million citations for biomedical literatre from MEDLINE life science journals, and online books. Citations may include links to full-text content from PubMed Center and publisher web sites. Here you can find clinical research abstracts on eating disorders as well as a variety of other medical/psychiatric problems.
AHRQ	Agency for Healthcare Research Quality	http://www.ahrq.gov/downloads/pub/evidence/pdf/eatingdisorders/eatdis.pdf	Review of evidence-based research.
EDRS	Eating Disorder Research Society	www.edresearchsociety.org	International organization of researchers that holds annual scientific meeting during which the most recent research can be presented and discussed.
Kantor & Kantor	Lisa Kantor	www.kantorlaw.net	Insurance litigation expert.
	Psych Appeal	www.psych-appeal.org	Mental health insurance advocacy (works with providers at patient request).
F.R.E.E.D. Foundation	Gail R. Schoenbach Foundation for Recovery and Elimination of Eating Disorders	www.freedfoundation.org	Advocacy, increase public awareness, raise funds and provide financial support for those who need treatment.
	Proud2BMe	www.proud2Bme.org	This site aims to counteract pro-anorexia and pro-bulimia websites.
MHA	Mental Health America	http://takeaction.mentalhealthamerica.net	Information on parity laws.
U.S. Dept. of Human Health Services (HHS)	HIPAA Laws	www.hhs.gov/ocr/privacy/hipaa/understanding/index.html	Understanding HIPAA restrictions.
	UC San Diego Eating Disorders Treatment and Research Program	http://eatingdisorders.ucsd.edu/	In addition to providing inpatient, intensive outpatient, and PHP program, the UCSD program offers a week-long intensive multi-family therapy program for anorexia

			sufferers and their families, using an evidence-based approach.
	University of Chicago Eating Disorders Program	http://psychiatry .uchicago.edu/re search/eatingDis ordersProgram.h tml	In addition to providing a variety of treatment programs, Dr. Daniel Le Grange and Dr. Eunice Chen are conducting a National Institute of Health funded research study designed to develop and refine a family-based treatment manual for young adults with Anorexia.
	Stanford University ED Treatment and Research Program	http://edresearc h.stanford.edu	This program is led by Dr. James Lock, to which Dr. Kathleen Kara Fitzpatrick lends her expertise. Their commitment to understanding and evaluating treatments through state-of-the-art research is evidenced by a number of important goals. They work to evaluate therapies and therapeutic outcomes as well as basic science at the level of brain functioning and imaging.
	Aimee Liu's website	www.gainingthet ruth.com	Author Aimee Liu's website, with information on her books and other resources on recovery.
CED	Center for Eating Disorders	www.center4ed.o rg	Outpatient treatment, education, support and referral services.
	The Bodywise Program	www.thebodywis eprogram.com	Treatment for recovery from compulsive eating and Binge Eating Disorder.
	National Eating Disorders	www.nationaleati ngdisorders.com	Link to numerous related websites.
	Behavior Tech	www.behaviortec h.org	This site provides information on CBT and DBT mindfulness training.
EDC	Eating Disorders Coalition	http://www.eati ngdisorderscoalit ion.org	Advocacy and political action, including seeking federal recognition of eating disorders as a public health priority.
	Dad Man	www.theDadMa n.com	Author Joe Kelly's website to promote the vital contribution of fathers to families, communities, organizations, work places, et al.
	Dads and Daughters with Eating Disorders	http://dad-eds.com/blog	Resource and support group for fathers of daughters with eating disorders.
AED	Academy for	www.aedweb.org	Global professional association

	Eating Disorders	/source/charter	committed to leadership in eating disorders research, education, treatment and prevention.
	The Anna Westin Foundation	Annawestin-foundation.org	The outrage at their daughter, Anna's, death and the outpouring of community support led Anna's family to establish The Anna Westin Foundation, a nonprofit organization formed to help others suffering directly or indirectly from eating disorders, and to provide education and information designed to prevent the development of anorexia and bulimia.
	Psychiatry Online	www.psychiatryonline.com/pracGuide/pracGuide-Topic_12aspx	2006 AOA Practice Guidelines for the Treatment of Patients with ED (third edition)

Residential Treatment Facilities in the U.S.

We recently read in the New York Times that there are 75 residential treatment facilities in the United States, the first of which was established in 1985. The majority of such facilities have come into existence since the beginning of this century. We searched a variety of websites in order to compile as complete a list as we could find. We apologize if any have been inadvertently omitted. Our list includes only 62.

	Name	State [City]
1	Anna Westin House	MN (St. Paul)
2	A Place of Hope	WA (Edmonds)
3	Avalon Hills	UT (Petersboro)
4	Bella Vita Bella Speranza	CA (Los Angeles)
5	Cambridge ED Ctr.	MA (Cambridge)
6	Casa Palmera	CA (Del MAR)
7	Castlewood	Missouri (St. Louis)
8	Canopy Cove	Florida (Tallahassee)
9	Carolina House	NC (Durham)
10	Center for Change	UT (Orem)
11	Center for Discovery	CA (Downey)
12	Center for	CA (Lakewood)

	Discovery	
13	Center for Discovery	CA (Whittier)
14	Center for Discovery	CA (Menlo Park)
15	Center for Discovery	WA (Redmond)
16	Oceanaire (CFD)	CA (Rancho Palos Verdes)
17	Oceanaire (CFD)	WA (Bellevue)
18	Oceanaire (CFD)	CA (Fremont)
19	Center for Hope of the Sierras	NV (Reno)
20	Eating Recovery Center	CO (Denver)
21	ED Network of MD	MD
22	Fairwinds	FL (Clearwater)
23	Harmony Place at St. Joseph's Villa	NY (Rochester)
24	Klarman ED Center at McLean Hospital (Harvard affiliate)	MA (Belmont)
25	Laureate	OK (Tulsa)
26	Laurel Hill Inn	
27	Lindner Center for Hope	OH (Cincinnati)
28	Linden Oaks	IL (Naperville)
29	Magnolia Creek	AL (Birmingham)
30	Montacatini	CA (Carlsbad)
31	Milestones	FL (Cooper City)
32	Mirasol	AZ (Tucson)
33	Monte Nido	CA (Malibu)
34	Monte Nido Vista	CA (Agoura Hills)
35	New Dawn	CA (San Francisco)
36	Oliver Pyatt	FL (Miami)
37	Park Nicolette Melrose Institute	MI
38	Puenta De Vida	CA (San Diego)
39	Rain Rock	OR (Eugene)
40	Rader Programs	CA (Ventura)
41	Reasons	CA (Pasadena)
42	Remuda Ranch	AZ (Chandler)
43	Rebecca's House	
44	Renfrew Center	PA (Philadelphia)
45	Renfrew Center	FL (Coconut Creek)
46	Renfrew Center	NJ (Ridgewood)

47	Renfrew Center	NY (New York)
48	Renfrew Center	PA (Philadelphia)
49	Renfrew Center	CT (Old Greenwich)
50	Renfrew Center	NC (Charlotte)
51	Renfrew Center	TN (Brentwood)
52	Renfrew Center	TX (Dallas)
53	Renfrew Center	MD (Bethesda)
54	Rogers Memorial Hospital	WI
55	Rosewood Ranch	AZ (north of Phoenix)
56	Selah House	IN (Anderson)
57	Sierra Tucson	AZ (north of Tucson)
58	Timberline Knolls	IL (Chicago)
59	Tapestry	NC (Brevard)
60	Turning Point	FL (Tampa)
61	Walden	MA (Waltham)
62	Wellspring Foundation	CT (Bethlehem)

People whose research it would be wise to become familiar with:

- Daniel Le Grange (University of Chicago)
- Walter Kaye (UC San Diego)
- Eunice Chen (University of Chicago)
- James Lock (Stanford University)
- Kathleen Kara Fitzpatrick (Stanford University)
- Janet Treasure (King's College London)
- Cynthia Bulik (University of North Carolina)
- James Greenblatt (Tufts Medical School)

Books to Read:

Gurze Books (www.bulimia.com) is a publishing company specializing in resources for eating disorders recovery. It was established when the owners co-wrote the book Bulimia: A Guide to Recovery, about the wife (Lindsey Cohn)'s, recovery from bulimia. They offer a bookstore of more than 300 handpicked titles, hundreds of articles, a directory of therapists, and listings of national organizations and treatment centers. They publish books on eating disorders, as well as a free eating disorder catalog, which includes titles from many other publishers. They also publish a bimonthly newsletter, which summarizes current research and treatment, and a monthly newsletter.

In addition to becoming familiar with Gurze Books, we recommend the following books, which we are listing under two main categories: Psycho-education, and Memoir. If you are on a budget and you don't mind buying used books, many of these, and others which we have yet to read, are available at amazon.com.

Psycho-educational titles:

(It is important to note the year in which it is published so that you can regard the information in its proper historical perspective.)

1. A Collaborative Approach to Eating Disorders, June Alexander and Janet Treasure PhD FRCP FRCPsych, eds. (2012)

2. The Treatment of Eating Disorders, A Clinical Handbook, Carlos Grilo PhD, James Mitchell MD, eds. (2010)

3. Answers to Anorexia: A Breakthrough Nutritional Treatment That Is Saving Lives, Dr. James Greenblatt (October, 2010)

4. Help Your Teenager Beat an Eating Disorder, James Lock MD PhD and Daniel Le Grange PhD (Jan 1, 2005)

5. Treatment Manual for Anorexia Nervosa: A Family Based Approach, James Lock MD and PhD, Daniel Le Grange PhD, W. Stewart Agras M.D. and Christopher Dare (Aug 29, 2002)

6. Skills-based Learning for Caring for a Loved One with an Eating Disorder: The New Maudsley Method, Janet Treasure, Grainne Smith and Anna Crane (July, 2007)

7. Eating Disorder Sourcebook, 3rd ed., Carolyn Costin, MA, MFT (2007)

8. 100 Q and A's About Eating Disorders, Carolyn Costin, MA, MFT (2007)

9. Take Charge of Your Child's Eating Disorder, Pamela Carlton, MD (December, 2006)

10. Demystifying Anorexia Nervosa: An Optimistic Guide to Understanding and Healing, Alexander Lucas, MD (February, 2004)

11. Unlocking the Mysteries of Eating Disorders: A Life-Saving Guide to Your Child's Treatment and Recovery, David Herzog, MD, Debra Franko, PhD, and Patti Cable (July, 2007)

12. Anatomy of Anorexia, Steven Levenkrom, PhD (2000)

13. It's Not About the Weight: Attacking Eating Disorders from the Inside Out, Susan Mendelsohn PsyD (2007)

14. Overcoming Anorexia Nervosa: A Self-Help Guide Using Cognitive Behavior Therapy, Christopher Freeman, MD PhD (2002)

15. Fasting Girls: The History of Anorexia Nervosa, Joan Jacobs Brumberg, PhD (1988)

16. It's Not Your Fault: Overcoming AN and BN through Biopsychiatry, Russell Marx, MD (April, 1991)

17. Surviving an Eating Disorder: Strategies for Family and Friends, 3rd Ed., Michele Siegel, PhD, Judith Brisman, MSW, Margot Weinshel, PhD (2009)

18. Eating with Your Anorexic: How My Child Recovered Through Family-based Therapy and Yours Can Too, Laura Collins (2005)

19. Eating By the Light of the Moon, Anita Johnston, PhD (1996)

20. The Golden Cage, Hilde Bruch, PhD (1978)

21. Eating Disorders – A Parents' Guide, 2nd ed., Dr. Rachel Bryant Waugh, PhD, and Bryan Lask, MD (June, 2004)

22. When Your Child Has an Eating Disorder: A Step-by-Step Workbook for Parents and Other Caregivers, Abigail H. Natenshon, MA, LCSW, GCFP (1999)

23. Anorexia and Bulimia in the Family: One Parent's Practical Guide to Recovery, by Grainne Smith

24. Dying To Please: Anorexia, Treatment and Recovery, Avis Rumney

25. Life Beyond Your Eating Disorder, Johanna Kandel, Founder and Executive Director, The Alliance for ED Awareness

26. Off the C.U.F.F.!!!!, Nancy Zucker, PhD, Duke University Medical Center (2004)

27. Treatment of Eating Disorders, A Clinical Handbook, by Carlos M. Grilo, PhD, and James E. Mitchell, MD (2011)

28. What Every Parent Needs to Know About Eating Disorders, Tonja Krautter

29. Inside Anorexia: The Experiences of Girls and Their Families, Christine Halse, Anne Honey and Desiree Boughtwood

Memoir Titles:

1. Next To Nothing: A Firsthand Account of One Teenager's Experience with an ED, Carrie Arnold (2007)

2. Running on Empty: A Diary of Anorexia and Recovery, Carrie Arnold (2004)

3. Anorexia: A Stranger in the Family, Katie Metcalf (2006)

4. Thin: A Memoir of Anorexia and Recovery, Grace Bowman (2008)

5. Kid Rex: The Inspiring True Account of a Life Salvaged from Anorexia, Despair and Dark Days in NYC, Laura Moisin (2008)

6. Life Without Ed, Jenni Schaefer

7. Andrea's Voice: Silenced by Bulimia, Doris Smeltzer

8. Gaining: The Truth About Life After Eating Disorders, Aimee Liu

9. Hungry: A Mother and Daughter Fight Anorexia, Sheila and Lisa Himmel

10. Anorexics on Anorexia, edited by Rosemary Shelley

11. <u>Stick Figure: A Diary of My Former Self</u>, Lori Gottleib

12. <u>Homesick: A Memoir of Family, Food, and Finding Hope</u>, Jenny Lauren (niece of Ralph Lauren)

13. <u>Going Hungry: Writers on Desire, Self-Denial, and Overcoming Anorexia</u>, edited by Kate Taylor

14. <u>Biting Anorexia</u>, Lucy Howard-Taylor

15. <u>Perfect: Anorexia and Me (Perfection was my disease… anorexia was my perfection)</u>, Emily Halban

16. <u>Unbearable Lightness</u>, by Portia De Rossi

17. <u>Brave Girl Eating</u>, by Harriet Brown

18. <u>My Kid is Back</u>, June Alexander and Professor Daniel Le Grange

19. <u>A Girl Named Tim</u>, by June Alexander

www.ingramcontent.com/pod-product-compliance
Lightning Source LLC
Chambersburg PA
CBHW072312290526
45794CB00002B/624